the
eczema
SOLUTION

the eczema SOLUTION

Sue Armstrong-Brown

First published in 2002 by Vermilion,
an imprint of Ebury Press
Random House Group
Random House
20 Vauxhall Bridge Road
London SW1V 2SA

www.rbooks.co.uk

Addresses for companies within
The Random House Group Limited can be found at:
www.randomhouse.co.uk/offices.htm

The Random House Group Limited Reg. No. 954009

A CIP catalogue record for this book
is available from the British Library

ISBN 9780091882846

Typeset by seagulls
Printed and bound in Great Britain by
CPI Antony Rowe, Chippenham, Wiltshire

The Random House Group Limited supports The Forest Stewardship
Council (FSC), the leading international forest certification organisation.
All our titles that are printed on Greenpeace approved FSC certified paper
carry the FSC logo. Our paper procurement policy can be found at:
www.rbooks.co.uk/environment

Although every effort has been made to ensure that the contents of this book
are accurate, it must not be treated as a substitute for qualified medical advice.
Always consult a qualified medical practitioner. Neither the Author nor the
Publisher can be held responsible for any loss or claim arising out of the use,
or misuse, of the suggestions made or the failure to take medical advice.

Illustrations on pages 16, 17, 28, 39, 47, 71, 76, 80 and 110 are reference:
Bridgett, C. Noren, P, & Staughton, R (1996), *Atopic skin disease: a manual for practitioners*. Wrightson Biomedical Publishing Ltd, Petersfield.

contents

Acknowledgements   viii

Foreword   ix

Chapter 1

Introduction   1

  Living with eczema   2

Chapter 2

Getting out of the downward spiral   10

  Atopy   10

  Acute and chronic eczema   12

  The vicious circle of chronic eczema   13

    Dry skin   13

    Eczematous skin   13

    Itching and scratching   14

    The vicious circle   15

  Treating each level of eczema   16

  Using this book   17

Chapter 3

Habit Reversal: registering the problem   20

  Logging your scratching   20

  Click!   22

  Recording the scratches   24

  Personal history   27

  Self-monitoring   27

    Eczema severity   28

    Old and new eczema   28

Distribution of eczema   29
Percentage of scratching coming from itch   29

Chapter 4
The Combined Approach: Levels 1 and 2   31
Emollients   33
Topical steroids   37
Mental state   40
Levels 1 and 2 Treatment Plan   43
Next appointment   44

Chapter 5
Habit Reversal: addressing the problem   46
ABC of scratching   47
Switching from scratching   48
Danger times   51
Self-prescription   53
What now?   54

Chapter 6
Habit Reversal: beating the problem   56
Eczema severity and distribution   57
Levels 1 and 2 Treatment review   57
Level 1: Emollients   58
Level 2: Steroids   58
Level 3 Treatment: Habit Reversal   59
Scratching frequency and cause   59
Troubleshooting   60
Focus times   61
What now?   64

Chapter 7

The healing curve   66

Eczema severity and distribution   67

Levels 1 and 2 Treatment review   67

    Level 1: Emollients   68

    Level 2: Steroids   68

Level 3 Treatment: Habit Reversal   69

The healing curve   70

Relapse recognition   72

    Stress   75

Chapter 8

Living without eczema   79

The convalescent phase   79

Complete healing   81

Living without eczema   85

    Vigilance and the Zap Pack   85

    Refresher courses   86

    If things go wrong: when to see your doctor   87

    Quality of life   88

Chapter 9

Frequently Asked Questions   90

Appendix 1

Topical Corticosteroids in common use   97

Appendix 2

Workbook   99

ACKNOWLEDGEMENTS

Lots of people helped to bring this book to life.

My family supported me through all the terrible years of severe eczema, and encouraged me to write this book to bring hope to others. The wonderful team at Chelsea and Westminster Hospital taught me to be free of eczema and gave me back my life. My agent, Judy Chilcote, was brave enough to take on an unknown author and from the moment I met her, wearing a Stars and Stripes sweater so I could recognise her from her accent, I knew she'd get the book to a publisher. My editor, Jacq Burns, brought her own brand of sympathy and personal involvement to the project. I'd like to thank Laura Taylor, Su-Lin Dow, Helen Weaving and Reggie Kandola for sharing their experiences of eczema and the Habit Reversal programme with me.

But most of all, I would like to thank Dr Chris Bridgett of Chelsea and Westminster Hospital, who helped and encouraged me every step of the way, unstintingly giving his time, expertise and advice. Without his support, this book would never have been written.

foreword

In the 1980's my old friend and colleague Dr Richard Staughton, Consultant Dermatologist at Westminster Hospital, heard a Swedish Dermatologist, Dr Peter Norén talk about a new and exciting approach to treating long-standing atopic eczema. Dr Norén had first reasoned that an established habit of rubbing and scratching skin, as often happens with atopic eczema, prevents treatment with creams from having the desired effect. He had then enlisted the help of a psychologist, who told him about a behaviour modification technique, *habit reversal*. Habit reversal was easy to learn, and proved effective in treating habitual scratching in atopic eczema. Research was published to show that combining habit reversal with creams was clearly superior to using creams on their own, when treating chronic atopic eczema.

So where did I come in? I was interested in how people with skin diseases could be helped psychologically. Dr Staughton told me he would like to make habit reversal available to his patients here in London, so we agreed to collaborate with Dr Norén. Very quickly it has become clear we are using a self-help treatment which is very effective indeed. So far we have taught the technique in our clinic, and have showed nurses and doctors how it can be taught not only in hospital clinics, but also in general practice. But there are so many people who could be helped, and it seemed important to find a way of making the treatment more generally available.

Then along came Sue Armstrong-Brown. We treated her eczema using Dr Norén's method, and as you can now read, she was so delighted by the results, she has written a book for others to read and benefit from her experience. If you have established chronic atopic eczema, and you are frustrated by the creams not working, then read this book. Discover how, by becoming your own expert, by understanding how to reverse the habit of rubbing and scratching, and by using the appropriate creams in the correct way you can clear your skin, and change your life! Instead of learning how to *Live with Eczema*, learn here how you can *Live without Eczema*.

DR CHRISTOPHER BRIDGETT
CONSULTANT PSYCHIATRIST
CHELSEA AND WESTMINSTER HOSPITAL, LONDON

chapter one
INTRODUCTION

At school it was the same old story: "Ooh she's got the lurgy"
or "Is it catching?"

This book is about getting rid of your chronic atopic eczema for
ever! The following chapters take you through a step-by-step
programme that will help you to learn about your eczema, how
to control it and finally to banish it. You will have clear, normal
skin, and will have learnt the techniques to ensure that it stays
that way.

I suffered from severe atopic eczema for years and had given
up hope of ever being free from it. Conventional treatments,
alternative therapies and periods in hospital had all failed to
control the condition. When I started this programme I was in a
very bad way, emotionally and physically. Four months later my
skin was better than it had been for over ten years. Now, when I
refer to having been ill, new acquaintances look at my skin and
do not believe me!

Terms for atopic eczema

People are often confused by the range of names for their skin condition, the most common being dermatitis and eczema. Below is a list of synonymous terms, all of which describe the same condition.

❑ Atopic eczema
❑ Atopic dermatitis
❑ Atopic skin disease
❑ Besnier's prurigo (the old name for the condition)

The programme has been developed by a group of dermatologists and psychologists in Sweden and England. It was originated by Dr Peter Noren, a Swedish dermatologist. Dr Richard Staughton, a British dermatologist, and Chris Bridgett, a psychiatrist, worked with Dr Noren to develop the programme for use in dermatology departments of British NHS hospitals. They also provide training for primary carers (GPs and nurse practitioners) at Chelsea and Westminster Hospital in London, some of whom are setting up their own eczema clinics based on this approach. However, there are over a million people in the UK who suffer from eczema, and who do not have access to this method of treatment. This book is for you.

Living with eczema

Those of us who have suffered with eczema know the traumas and problems all too well. But we sometimes feel that the people who should be helping us to cope with it don't really understand it themselves. An example that springs to mind is a conversation I had with a young nurse, the second time I was

Types of eczema

As well as atopic eczema, there are several other types of eczema (or dermatitis).

❑ Atopic: the subject of this book

❑ Seborrheic: associated with the natural oily secretions from the skin

❑ Occupational: caused by contact with particular allergens and irritants

❑ Varicose or Gravitational: associated with poor circulation

❑ Discoid: predominantly in the elderly

hospitalized for eczema. She had been working in different departments all round the hospital to gain experience in various types of nursing, and I asked her which she had enjoyed most. She said that she preferred the oncology and cardiac wards to the general medical ward that I was on, because 'after all, you aren't really ill, are you?'.

It is just this type of comment that leads many people with eczema to feel that they should simply keep quiet and put up with it. After all, it isn't life threatening. And we are often told that the condition can't be cured, and all we can do is *learn to live with it*. But who wants to live with eczema?

So we turn to alternative therapies. There are certainly a lot to choose from, and some of them do help. But in the long run many sufferers lose faith in ever finding a way to get rid of their eczema. We can't get excited about new treatments because experience has taught us that in the long run they don't really work. And we don't believe people who give us advice because, after all, they don't know what it's really like.

This chapter is to demonstrate to you that I do know exactly what having eczema is like. I am now 34 and have had eczema since I was six weeks old. All through my childhood I had flare-ups, which were relatively quickly controlled by steroid creams. At first I had the classic infantile eczema distribution: in the flexures (folds of knees and elbows), the wrists and neck, and the corners of my mouth. I don't actually remember being much troubled by my skin as a child, although my mother tells me that I was a horrendously grouchy baby. I suppose I was comparatively lucky in that I did not develop asthma as a child (that came later!). The two conditions, together with hay fever, are often linked. Asthma receives a much higher profile and more informed treatment than eczema, something which eczema carers and patients, and the National Eczema Society, are working to change.

By the time I was 14 the skin on my trunk and arms was included in the flare-ups, although in between these times it would still clear completely. When I left school at 18 I experienced my first prolonged period of acute eczema, which ended in my being hospitalized for two-and-a-half weeks. I still remember the shock when the doctor told me that it wouldn't clear on its own, and that I would have to come into hospital. I hadn't really thought of eczema as an illness in that way before. It had always been something like flu; unpleasant and unpredictable, but not particularly serious.

That period in hospital gave me a year of almost completely clear skin. But after that things went downhill rapidly, and when I was 21 I was back in hospital again for another week with *eczema herpeticum*. This is an especially foul variation, where eczematous skin gets infected with the cold sore virus. It started under my arm of all places, and spread rapidly across my chest and side. It hurts terribly and is spread very quickly by the inevitable scratching. You may already know that atopic people are often more than usually susceptible to many infections, and this is a particularly nasty consequence. Ever since that first outbreak I've had to look out for relapses, although thankfully they were never as bad again.

My skin never really cleared up after that. It was better when I left hospital, but it soon came back and I struggled with it through the rest of my supposedly carefree student career. As I became better informed I started worrying about the side-effects of long-term steroid use. You've probably heard all the same horror stories I did: that it stunts your growth; damages the skin permanently; causes dermatitis on healthy skin; and seems to become gradually less and less effective and you end up using more and more, becoming, in effect, a steroid junkie.

I tried to cut down the amount I was using, which of course only made my skin worse, and I started the search for alternative cures. I probably tried every one in the book. My family was wonderfully supportive, encouraging me and helping me to pay for expensive treatments, and coming up with suggestions them-selves. I tried herbalism, hypnotherapy, acupuncture, shiatsu, radiology, magnetology, exclusion diets, meditation, creative visualization, aromatherapy, reflexology, Chinese herbs, homeo-pathy ... and probably a few more.

Most of them seemed to help at first. I still don't know whether this was an illusion because I so much wanted them to work, or if feeling better because I was doing something positive helped, or indeed if the treatments were effective to some degree. Chinese herbs and homeopathy both had real effects that lasted for weeks. But eventually I had to acknowledge that I was persevering with them because I didn't want to admit that they had helped as much as they were going to.

I don't want to dismiss complementary therapies completely here as several did wonders in combating the emotional and psychological repercussions of having severe eczema. Particularly good were my sessions with a very perceptive homeopathist, who helped me to recognize the damage that my skin was doing to my personality and to try to repair it. I am also lucky enough to have an aunt qualified in reflexology and the soothing treatments she gave me calmed me down and reduced the insomnia that so often accompanies inflamed skin.

I remember when it first occurred to me that I might not get better. I was 22. I had always thought in terms of *when* my skin cleared. When I have clear skin I'll be able to get a tan/wear black/go to the gym/sleep properly/be more confident. But suddenly it dawned on me that I might always have eczema. I might never get rid of it. I might have it for ever. It was a terrible thought, and I actively avoided thinking about it for months. But it gradually insinuated its way into my consciousness, and I believed it. That started a very bad period for me. My skin continued to get worse and I became depressed.

For the next six years I blamed everything that went wrong in my life on having eczema. I watched it creep over the whole of my body, and it was actually a relief when it reached the soles of my feet. It couldn't spread any further after that. I went into hospital for a fortnight again and was treated with steroid injections and bandages, but it was back within three weeks of being discharged.

My skin was so dry that it came off in sheets. I woke up every morning looking as if I'd been rolled in oat flakes. I had to put on emollients all over every couple of hours during the day and night. I dreaded being anywhere with dark carpets or furniture, because it would look as if it had snowed around me if I stayed there for any length of time. Whenever I went to the lavatory at work to apply cream the floor looked as if someone had dropped a bag of flour. After I noticed white footprints leading out of the bathroom and along the hall I started going through a humiliating ritual of sweeping the floor with a wad of toilet paper, to clean up after myself.

I hated the summer because when I got hot the sweat stung, and flies were attracted to my weeping scratches. I couldn't wear short sleeves or skirts or shorts. I hated rain because it stung my raw scalp and hands. I hated cold weather, because I was usually freezing; my inflamed erythrodermic skin pumped out so much heat that I was hot to the touch but shivering with cold.

I couldn't wear dark colours because they showed the skin flakes. I couldn't wear lightweight materials or pale colours because they tore when I scratched and the bloodstains showed through. I saved up new clothes and wouldn't wear them because it would spoil them. My hairstyles were designed to cover as much of my hairline, forehead, ears and neck as poss-ible. Make-up and jewellery were impossible.

Every movement hurt. My skin lost all its elasticity. When I stood up from a chair I had to hobble for a minute while the skin on my legs grudged its way into a new shape. Straightening my elbows or knees gave me 'elephant skin' wrinkles for inches around each joint. Moving suddenly sometimes made my skin split painfully. I would save up tasks that involved moving until I had enough to make it worth the pain of action.

I scratched so much and so hard that my nails would split across. Chunks of skin would get rammed down inside them, setting off infections with a painful build-up of pus and pressure behind my nails. I had to psyche myself up every day to get into a bath or shower, bracing myself against the sting of water on my mangled skin. I hated my body and was obsessed with it – sometimes looking at my seeping, flaking, red, swollen and encrusted skin would revolt me so much I felt sick.

My work and social relationships suffered. Being upset over my skin had evolved into being clinically depressed. I was always exhausted and craving sleep. I didn't want to go out or talk to people. I was a nervous wreck, jumping if someone spoke behind me and bursting into tears if I dropped a pencil. Simple tasks became a huge struggle.

The crunch came when my parents came to stay with me for a weekend. I was so frazzled after the morning ritual of getting up and dealing with all the deterioration during the night that making them a morning cup of tea proved to be beyond me. I couldn't tear my hands away from scratching for long enough to fill up the kettle. My parents were terribly upset and ganged up with my boyfriend to make me go to my GP and ask for help.

This wasn't as simple as it sounds! I had created the illusion of coping that a lot of eczema sufferers have, putting up a smoke screen of jokes and bravado because they don't know what else to do. I had been refusing my GP's various offers to refer me to a dermatologist for years because I didn't think there was any point. After all, I had already been hospitalized three times and in the long run it hadn't done any good. I just collected repeat prescriptions for steroids and emollients and pretended that everything was fine.

Going to my GP and admitting that I wasn't coping was very difficult. In fact, I just went to pieces and cried all over the poor man until *he* told *me* that I wasn't coping! I asked to be referred to the Chelsea and Westminster Hospital in London, because I had heard of their progressive treatment programme for eczema patients. My GP wrote to the local Health Authority to get permission to refer me out of the area and I duly presented myself at the Dermatology Clinic three months later when my appointment came through.

I can honestly say that this appointment changed my life.

CASE STUDY

Su-Lin is 37. Looking at pictures of herself as a child, she says 'I have my hands behind my back, or one finger in the palm of the other; I was always scratching.' After having her own children, her eczema ran out of control. 'It was all over my face and really disfiguring. I wanted to avoid people... it became a third unspoken presence in a conversation. On the one hand people studiously wanted to avoid the issue, and on the other they wanted to say "what happened to your face?"'

Her work as an actress suffered, limiting her to voice work and radio. When it was really bad, she only felt comfortable walking around on winter nights; the cold took away the itchy burning feeling and the darkness helped cover her face.

The most important thing that the Habit Reversal programme taught Su-Lin was that she had some control in the management of her skin. 'The system made me examine how natural it was for me to instinctively scratch. I would say that it provided the first real benchmark enabling me to help myself.'

chapter two
GETTING OUT OF THE DOWNWARD SPIRAL

I had become an eczema person and couldn't see myself without it. I didn't believe I could ever be completely well.

If you follow the programme described in this chapter, using the steps set out in the rest of the book, you will discover how you too can live without eczema. But first of all you need to understand eczema, what it is and why it is so difficult to control and treat effectively.

Atopy

Atopy means 'strange disease', which should give you an idea of how difficult it is to define. The term was coined in the 1920s to describe people who are prone to eczema, asthma,

---

How common is atopy?

25–30 per cent of the general population is atopic.

5–15 per cent of school children have atopic eczema.

2–10 per cent of adults have atopic eczema.

---

and hay fever. There is no one hard and fast diagnostic symptom for atopy.

We are often told that eczema cannot be cured, but really it is *atopy* that cannot be cured. People who are atopic have a greater chance of suffering from eczema, as well as the related conditions of asthma and hay fever. Atopy is something that you are born with, and you can't change it. But the important thing to remember is this: atopy does not mean a life sentence of eczema. Plenty of atopic people never develop eczema, or grow out of it. You will always be atopic. But you don't always have to have eczema.

Diagnosing atopic eczema

Although it is not possible to pin atopic eczema down to an exact set of symptoms, there are some general signs which help to identify it. Ask yourself these questions:

1   Do I have an itchy skin condition?
2   Do I have a history of itchy rashes, especially in skin creases?
3   Do I have a history of asthma or hay fever?
4   Has my skin been generally dry over the last year?
5   Do I have a visible rash, especially in skin creases?
6   Did I start having itchy rashes before I was two?
7   Has my condition been diagnosed as atopic eczema by a specialist?
8   Do I have a family history of eczema, asthma or hay fever?

If you said 'yes' to no. 1 and any three of the others, you can be diagnosed as having atopic eczema – check with your doctor.

Acute and chronic eczema

If you think back over the way your skin has behaved during the last few months you will probably remember periods when your skin was fairly stable and times when it flared up and got worse. The flare-ups are periods of acute eczema. These often happen in response to an external stimulus, such as a change in lifestyle, a source of stress or sorrow, catching a bug, feeling tired, or coming into contact with something to which you are allergic. Acute eczema can appear and vanish within a few days.

Chronic eczema is the bit left over when the acute eczema has subsided, the background skin condition that doesn't change. The level of chronic eczema varies from person to person. Your skin might clear except for a few patches that are always there, or you might always have eczema all over, with the difference between acute and chronic just a matter of severity. Either way, you will have the same pattern of ongoing chronic eczema with occasional blips of acute eczema.

Acute eczema can be dealt with using emollients and steroids, and it always responds to the right treatment. Chronic eczema is much more difficult to shift. This programme deals with how to get rid of the chronic eczema altogether. Your background skin condition will get better and better, until there is no chronic eczema at all. At the same time the blips of acute eczema will get less and less severe, and will be easier and easier to control.

As you are atopic you will always be susceptible to future attacks of acute eczema, but don't worry, they will never be as bad as they are now, and at the end of this programme you will know how to deal with them almost before they begin. We will come back to this topic in a later chapter.

The vicious circle of chronic eczema

When thinking about chronic eczema it is easiest to break it down into three levels and consider each one separately. The programme works by addressing each one of these factors with a different treatment, so it makes sense to think about them one at a time. The three levels are:

❏ dry skin
❏ eczema and itch
❏ scratching.

DRY SKIN

Many people with dry skin don't have eczema, but eczematous skin is always dry. The drying is caused by body fluids evaporating from the skin's surface too quickly. This is because skin with eczema is much more porous than healthy skin. It is a less effective barrier against moisture loss, and so the skin dries out faster. Dry skin is characterized by a taut, non-elastic feeling and by the presence of white flakes of dead skin cells. But the main problem for people with eczema is that dry skin is itchy skin.

ECZEMATOUS SKIN

There are several elements to eczematous skin. It becomes puffy and inflamed. The skin develops little fluid-filled vesicles, like bubbles, which weaken its structure. Blood vessels in the lower layers of the skin (the dermis) swell, and blood cells that fight infection migrate into the skin, causing redness and itch. Normal cell growth in the epidermis (outer skin layer) speeds up, causing cells to pile up and thicken the skin. The cells are smaller and weaker than healthy skin cells, and the lubricating liquid between the cells, which helps make normal skin flexible and waterproof, is disrupted. Older cells build up on the skin's surface, because the biological 'glue' that holds them together stops breaking down and allowing the cells to be gradually shed. This results in a thick layer of dead dry skin at the top of the epidermis.

ITCHING AND SCRATCHING

The first point to make here is that there is a difference between itching and scratching. Itching is a feeling while scratching is a behaviour. This is an important distinction to get on board, because we will come back to it later in the programme.

Scratching is a natural response to an itch or irritation. It is a reflex action, something that you don't always need to think about before you do it. It can often be automatic. For example, if you get a mosquito bite, often the first time you notice it is when you find yourself scratching it. Doctors have recently discovered that there are special nerves to sense itching, as well as those that sense temperature, pressure and pain.

Scratching is what makes the difference between acute and chronic eczema. Without scratching, chronic eczema cannot exist.

Skin with chronic eczema is unevenly thickened, with a rough, irregular appearance. This is called lichenification, because it can look similar to lichen growing on a tree or rock. It is due to the disruption of the epidermis that results from the continuous scratching of the sufferer. If healthy skin that has never had eczema is continually scratched it will develop the uneven appearance of skin with chronic eczema. If the scratching is stopped the skin recovers, and returns to its healthy, regular structure. Doctors have experimentally demonstrated this using scratching machines to constantly scratch a small area of non-eczematous skin. The skin then reacts by becoming lichenified, and recovers when the machine is stopped. Scratching also tears the skin and makes it more vulnerable to infection and further inflammation. It probably drives allergens to which you are sensitive into the skin as well.

How the damage is caused varies. Scratching is usually done with the fingernails. But rubbing skin on skin, such as with the palm of your hand, or clothes on skin, using the friction caused by the roughness of the fabric, is also damaging. So is picking. There is a wonderful range of scratching techniques out there, involving objects (hair brushes, forks, rivets on jeans, towels) or even someone else! The doctors who developed this programme say that they are continually astonished by the variety of scratching methods their patients tell them about. I even used to scald my hands under the hot water tap under the pretext of washing them to soothe an itch. When you come to follow this treatment programme even touching will count.

THE VICIOUS CIRCLE

The three elements of chronic eczema form a vicious circle. Each one makes the others worse, and the sufferer goes into a downward spiral of inflamed, dry, scratched and damaged skin. The inflammation is itchy and makes the skin dry, which makes it even itchier. Together they cause scratching, which makes the eczema worse, which makes the skin drier, which makes it itchier, and so on and so on. Eventually, scratching becomes habitual.

Habitual scratching develops through several stages. The normal response to an itch, scratching, becomes repetitive, because the skin is often itchy. Any repetitive behaviour can become a habit and, at least partially, unconscious. Thus, awareness of the behaviour is decreased. At the same time the scratching becomes linked to circumstances, situations and activities other than the original stimulus (in this case, itch). This is called generalization. In the end, scratching can be triggered by lots of different things or situations (as well as itch), and you may be scratching automatically almost all the time.

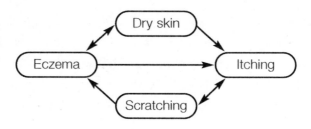

Figure 1: The vicious circle of chronic eczema

Treating each level of eczema

Conventionally, treatments have been based around managing dry skin, eczema and itch. The dryness is treated with emollients. The eczema is treated with steroids. Acute eczema responds well to this approach but in chronic eczema the scratching has become so well established that the skin never recovers. This is why we so often hear that there is no cure for eczema.

But there is a cure. It just involves dealing with the scratching as well as the dryness and the inflammation. 'Oh, simple!' I expect you're saying. 'Just stop scratching. Why haven't I thought of that before?'.

This is exactly the point of the whole programme. You can't just 'stop' scratching. You've probably tried for years; I know I did. Well-meaning people telling you to stop and that you're only making it worse don't help either; this only adds to the feeling that it's all your own fault.

Your scratching has become a habitual behaviour. At the moment you can no more stop it than you can stop, say, liking chocolate. This is why you need to relearn your response to itching. By following the programme set out here you will first understand when and why you scratch, then regain control over your scratch response, and finally you will replace it with a new, safe, response. This whole procedure is called **Habit Reversal**.

At the same time as Habit Reversal, you will be reviewing your usual treatments for the other two levels of the vicious circle, and refining them to make them as effective as possible. This programme works by addressing the eczema on all three levels simultaneously, taking away all of the causes of chronic eczema. It is called the **Combined Approach** to treating eczema, because it combines conventional treatments for Levels 1 and 2 (emollients and steroids) with Habit Reversal for Level 3.

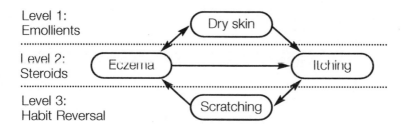

Figure 2: The Combined Approach:
treating all the levels of chronic eczema

Using this book

This book is structured to take you through the programme as if you were attending a series of visits with a doctor. Each chapter is one 'appointment'. There is nothing to stop you from reading it all through before you start, but I recommend that you do not. There is a danger that you might read through the whole programme, put the book down, and think, 'right, I'll go and do that then'. If you do, you won't be following the important step-by-step structure that has been specifically developed to address the fundamental biological and psychological causes of atopic eczema, and you might not master the Habit Reversal that is central to the programme.

The steps are all deceptively simple, but in practice they are much more demanding than they appear. So to give yourself the best chance, let the book set your pace. You can set aside one hour a week to read the next chapter and start the next step. You will feel a real sense of achievement as your skin gets better, your scratching comes under control, and you can see the light at the end of the tunnel: the prospect of living without eczema.

Points to remember

1 The three levels of chronic eczema are:
   ❑ dry skin
   ❑ eczema and itch
   ❑ scratching.
2 Without scratching, chronic eczema cannot exist.
3 This programme works by addressing chronic atopic eczema on all three levels simultaneously, dealing with all of the causes of chronic eczema. All three levels must be treated together. They are all equally important.

CASE STUDY

As a child, Reggie threw himself into sport to escape from the eczema that affected his schooldays. When he reached his 20s it began to wreak major damage – not just on his skin, but on his whole life. 'It was the worst eczema I'd ever seen, on anyone, let alone myself – and I'd been going to eczema clinics all my life,' he remembers. Reggie started drinking a bottle of vodka a night, just to try to sleep, and took up smoking – a far cry from the keen sportsman he had been. 'I was very low. I lost my sense of self – I was turning up at work with huge scratch wounds in my neck, and being sent away.' The turning point came when his doctors taught him about eczema. 'No one had even told me what type of eczema I had before, let alone what the steroids were doing.' Reggie, now 27, says that the most important process for him was education. 'I learnt about my skin, and was introduced to a new philosophy about controlling it.' The end of the process was Habit Reversal, which gave Reggie back the discipline that severe eczema had driven from his life. He threw himself into the programme, making notes and developing his own ideas. 'The discipline of logging my scratching bought me back to the person that I used to be: sporty and organised.' His attitude changed and he started to look forward. Now, two months after completing the programme, Reggie is a different person. 'I'm so thankful that my life is under control again.'

chapter three
HABIT REVERSAL: REGISTERING THE PROBLEM

*Once I went shopping, and someone refused to put change
into my hand. I remember it was all scaly and bandaged,
and they looked at me and put the money on the counter.
I felt terrible.*

We have already established that no amount of emollient or
steroid will get rid of chronic eczema while your skin is still being
damaged by scratching. You know you are scratching too much.
So the first question is this: exactly how much is too much? Your
behaviour has become a habit, and largely unconscious. In order
to change it you have to make it conscious.

Logging your scratching

First you need some equipment: a hand logger or tally counter.
Get one of these as soon as possible. You can buy them from
stationers and some sports shops for around £11 – details oppo-
site*. Or you can keep a notepad and pencil with you at all times
and keep a gate tally; not as easy as using a logger so do try to
get one if you can. If you have access to the internet, a quick

search will bring up several sites where you can order your counter: Acumen Books site (see below) has several types from £5–£10, including one you can strap round your wrist like a watch. It doesn't matter which type you get – choose whichever suits your budget and your sense of style.

Over the next week you are going to use your counter or notepad to log how many times you scratch in a day. Do this by clicking the counter (push the button on the top) or making a pencil mark every time you finish a scratch. Count each scratching episode as one scratch, rather than each backwards-and-forwards scratching motion, or you'll be up in the thousands within an hour. If you use two hands, for example during a concerted attack on both shins, that counts as two scratches, so click twice!

You also need to log times when you aren't *technically* scratching, but are still damaging or causing friction to your skin. This includes rubbing (even if it is gentle), scraping against something, picking (even if it is just to get rid of dry skin), and any other particular ritual you have developed. I'm sure you know the sort of thing I mean! (One of my favourite 'I'm not really scratching, honest' rituals, during boring periods of standing around waiting for laboratory experiments to finish, was to lean against a ridged radiator and then sway from side to side against the ridges. The excuse was that I was just trying to keep warm, but I could keep it up for hours and eventually the whole of my back would be completely raw. That's scratching!)

---

* **Places to buy your Hand Tally Counter** High Street stationers: Rymans sell them for around £11, and Staples will order them for you for the next day, at £15. Countersales UK Ltd: Call 0113 228 0059 or visit the website http://www.hand-tally.com. Prices are now £8.45 ex VAT for one counter. Postage is included. Road Runners: Call 0208 882 2749. They sell plastic hand tallies for around £11 plus VAT, postage and packing (ref: CA179). Acumen Books: website http://www. a-b.co.uk/amendex.htm sell a range of counters.

Choose your start day, and make sure you have your logger with you at all times. The easiest ways are to wear it on a cord around your neck, under your top if you don't want to be too conspicuous, or in the pocket of a garment you wear all day (not a jacket that you take off and leave somewhere). You must always have the logger on you for two reasons:

1 You won't remember to update it accurately later.
2 The point of this exercise is to register *when* you scratch, *as* you are doing it. Clicking the logger immediately after each scratch is the best way to register it, not only as a number in the day's total but also in your own mind: it makes it conscious.

Remember:

Always have your logger with you, and always log each scratch immediately. For this exercise, don't try to avoid scratching.
Scratching = rubbing
         = picking
         = touching.

Click!

At first you might have to concentrate to remember to log each scratch. Your scratching is habitual, and often you might be completely unaware that you are scratching. This is where enlisting the support of those around you comes in. Ask your friends and family to help remind you when you need to click your logger. Be careful; it is important to get the approach right here. In the past, every time someone told you to 'stop scratching' (which must have happened millions of times over the years) it sent a negative message that you were doing something wrong, even though you couldn't help it. Now, instead, ask them just to say 'click!' to you if they see you scratching. This just lets you know that you're doing it, and reminds you that when you stop you should log your scratch. Get others trained now, as this will come in very handy later in the programme!

It sounds minor but this really is a very important point, so forgive me for going on about it. Other people's reactions contribute a lot to your state of mind. The feeling of being out of control, ruled by your skin, is a familiar one to many people with chronic eczema. As a child you may have been told that scratching was 'nasty' or 'naughty', and as adults we still feel rather the same thing. Yet you still scratch, which often makes you feel guilty, weak or dirty. When other people notice, and tell you to stop, it compounds the negative feelings.

This programme is all about regaining control over your skin. We have no room for negative, out of control feelings here! It is vital that those close to you understand this. You can choose how much you want to explain – you could even ask them to read this chapter. Alternatively, just ask them to remind you that you're scratching by saying 'click' (nicely), and to leave the rest to you.

It is worth remembering that people who care about you probably feel quite upset and frustrated themselves when you scratch, because they can see the damage it does and that it distresses you. They may be relieved to have something to do which actually contributes to the programme, rather than feeling like a constant nagger.

I was lucky enough to have very supportive friends and family when I followed the programme, and they all did their bit with gusto. I remember the huge sense of relief the first time I was scratching, guiltily and frenziedly, while watching television, and instead of a 'stop scratching' or a slap on the wrist I just got a gentle 'click!'. All the external pressure was off – all I had to do was say 'thank you' and, without urgency, click my logger.

Obviously, you won't want all and sundry monitoring whether or not you have used your logger. I suggest you only involve those who would be commenting (telling you not to scratch) anyway, or those whom you feel comfortable about including. After a few days it will become more automatic, and you will find yourself reaching for your logger as soon as you stop scratching.

Whatever you do, don't worry about trying to stop scratching earlier in order to get to your logger, or even preventing yourself from scratching at all to keep the logger count down. At this stage we are just assessing what your normal scratching pattern is like, and raising your awareness of it.

Remember:

Ask your family and friends never to tell you not to scratch, but to remind you to register the scratch on your logger by saying 'click!'.

Recording the scratches

Find *Chart 1: Registration* in the Workbook (see page 99) and fill it in with the day's total; then reset the logger to zero by turning the knob on the side. You should then immediately start registering scratches for the next day's total.

It is up to you when to start your new day's count. After my first day I realized that there was no point in writing down a total when I went to bed and starting again in the morning because I was scratching so much when awake during the night, and these scratches were not being counted. So I kept the logger beside my

Scratching times

Most people have particular situations when they scratch most. Here are some typical ones:
❏ Getting dressed
❏ On the phone
❏ In the toilet
❏ While reading or writing
❏ Watching television
❏ Getting ready for bed
❏ In bed

bed within easy clicking reach, and wrote down the total first thing in the morning. However, don't worry about the scratching you do in your sleep – this doesn't count.

You will probably be absolutely horrified by the totals. What did you get? Don't panic! They may seem outrageously high, but just carry on clicking and recording your normal scratching pattern through the week. Some people log 60 scratches a day, and others with equally bad eczema log over 1000. It all depends on how you define 'one scratch'. In fact, the totals are not really that important. What matters is the way that they change through the programme. Be consistent in how you log a scratch, and don't try to avoid scratching. Just allow registration to make yourself more aware of when you do it.

When you write down each day's total, think back over the day. What were the most scratchy times? You did not scratch at a constant rate over the whole day. There were probably some periods where you were constantly scratching and clicking the logger. Note down the most scratchy times for each day on the form. There is an example of a completed chart below. We are not worrying about the last line, 'percentage of scratching coming from itch', just yet.

Remember:

Write down each day's total and the times when you scratched most, then reset the logger and start clicking the next day's scratches.

Chart 1: Registration – example

Day	**Friday**	**Saturday**
Total scratches	**682**	**597**
Times when I scratched most today		
1	**In the shower**	**Getting dressed**
2	**Getting dressed**	**Doing housework**
3	**On the phone**	**Getting ready to go out in the evening**
4	**Looking for a file**	**In the car**
5	**Getting ready for bed**	**Getting ready for bed**

Personal history

It is a good idea to spend some time this week taking stock of how your eczema has developed since when you first had it, until you reached the stage you are at now. If you were doing this programme in a hospital clinic, the doctor or nurse practitioner would take down the history of your eczema. You may have already given a history to a doctor, either a GP or a specialist you have been referred to.

Chart 2: History of eczema (see page 100) sets out the most important areas of your eczema's history that you should cover. Fill it in, but do not feel limited by it. You may want to write down the story of your eczema instead, going into much more detail about how it has developed, what affects it, and the impact it has had on your life. It is a useful way of reviewing everything that has happened, and helps you to focus on what, specifically, has been going on and what you might want to bear in mind during this programme. It can also be quite a therapeutic experience.

Self-monitoring

Self-monitoring is an essential characteristic of this programme. Monitor your scratching as set out above, recording how often and when you scratch. *Chart 3: Eczema review* (see page 103) is a chart that you will keep coming back to throughout the programme. It is a table of different measures of the state of your skin, which you will fill in every couple of weeks as you go along. There are three further measures:

❏ eczema severity scale from 0–10
❏ percentage of old versus new eczema
❏ distribution of eczema.

ECZEMA SEVERITY

The eczema severity scale is an informal way of assessing how good or bad your eczema is. We measure it on a subjective scale from 0 to 10. Think about the worst your eczema has ever been: where it was; what it looked like; how it felt. This is 10. Perfect skin is zero. How does your skin score at the moment?

OLD AND NEW ECZEMA

The difference between acute and chronic eczema was described in Chapter 2. Acute eczema is the new eczema that appears in flare-ups and then subsides. Chronic eczema is the bit left over after the acute eczema has gone, the old patches that almost never clear up. The combination of acute and chronic eczema varies from person to person, and changes over time with an individual person. How much of your eczema is new, having appeared over the last ten days or so? How much is old, long-standing eczema that has been around for months or years? Try to give a score for

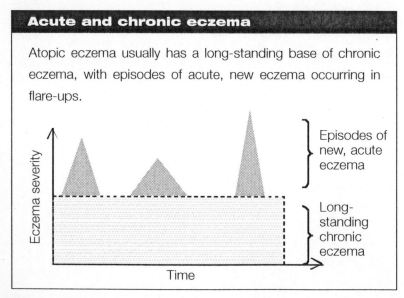

Acute and chronic eczema

Atopic eczema usually has a long-standing base of chronic eczema, with episodes of acute, new eczema occurring in flare-ups.

Episodes of new, acute eczema

Long-standing chronic eczema

Eczema severity

Time

the amount of your eczema that is old, chronic eczema (for example, 70 per cent of my eczema is old eczema).

DISTRIBUTION OF ECZEMA

Think about where your eczema is. Are some areas better than others, or even clear? Is your eczema restricted to patches of various sizes on particular parts of your body? Common areas for bad eczema include exposed body parts; bits that you can reach easily or dry out fast, such as hands, wrists, ankles, ears and shoulders. Note down the worst affected areas, and where the rest is.

Chart 4: Body map (see page 104) is a plan of a body, seen from the back and the front. Using a pencil, shade in the areas where your eczema is, with darker shading or cross-hatching, or a different colour, to differentiate the worst areas from the rest. This way you have a map of where your eczema is at the beginning of the programme. You may want to make copies of this chart, so that you can make several maps as you go through the programme. This is another way of recording your progress, as well as showing the areas that clear most quickly and the ones that prove more difficult to shift.

PERCENTAGE OF SCRATCHING
COMING FROM ITCH

In Chapter 2 we covered the difference between itching and scratching, establishing that itching is a sensation while scratching is a behaviour. Scratching usually occurs in response to an itch, but in people with chronic eczema the reaction may have generalized to a variety of stimuli, and may be partly unconscious. Over the last week how much of your scratching was directly as a result of feeling an itch?

Look at your most scratchy times on Chart 1. Were you scratching a lot because you were very itchy? Or do you just seem to scratch a lot in those situations? Most people find that a relatively low proportion of their scratching is actually coming from itch, although quite often a non-itchy scratch can then cause the skin to start itching, provoking further scratching. Try to give your scratching a score (for example, 25 per cent of my scratching is coming from itch).

You might also want to think about your scratching itself. How do you do it? Do you always scratch with your fingernails, or do you have other favourite techniques? How do you feel when you are scratching? How do you feel afterwards? How do other people react when you scratch?

See you next week!

Points to remember

1   Always have your logger with you, and always log each scratch immediately. Don't try to avoid scratching. Scratching = rubbing
    = picking
    = touching.

2   Ask your family and friends never to tell you not to scratch, but to remind you to register the scratch on your logger by saying 'click!'.

3   Write down each day's total and the times when you scratched most, then reset the logger and start clicking the next day's scratches.

chapter four

THE COMBINED APPROACH: LEVELS 1 AND 2

When other workmates used to sneak away for a cigarette,
I used to sneak away to the bathroom for a good scratch.

If everything has gone to plan you will have achieved a lot in the week between reading the last chapter and starting this one. You should have:

❏ trained your friends and family to remind you of when you're scratching by saying 'click';
❏ logged your scratching for seven days;
❏ noticed when you scratch the most during the day, and thought about why;
❏ completed a written record of your totals and pattern over the week by filling in *Chart 1: Registration;*
❏ completed a history of your eczema, either in *Chart 2* or as your own written story;
❏ started a system of self-monitoring in *Chart 3*, by scoring your eczema on how severe it is at the moment, how much of your eczema is old or new, and where it is.

If things have gone well, you will have learned more about your skin and your scratching in the last week than you have for a long time!

So now it is time to look at the first two treatment levels of the Combined Approach. These are Level 1: dry skin, which is treated with emollients, and Level 2: eczema and itching, which are treated with steroids. You must get appropriate treatment at these two levels in order to have the best chance of complete success with Level 3: scratching, which is treated with Habit Reversal.

The first thing to do is to enlist the support of your doctor. This could be your GP or, if you already attend a skin clinic, you could discuss the programme with your dermatologist.

Just let me just say a word of warning here. If you are already using emollients and steroids, and are thinking of skipping this step, think again. Perhaps you have been battling for years to reduce the amount of steroid you use, possibly with the usual cautious advice from your doctor. Perhaps you are simply fed up with conventional treatments and would rather go straight to the novel part of this programme. I do sympathize; I was completely nonplussed by conventional treatments when I started this programme. However, if this is how you feel, then please read the rest of this chapter through and have another think. It explains why you need to pay close attention to which steroids and emollients you use, and how you and your doctor will vary them according to the condition of your skin. To keep on trucking with the same old stuff you have always used may be completely inappropriate for you as you go through this programme. It was developed for use in hospital clinics, with a specialist to guide patients through every step. Only recently has it been considered as a treatment for nurses and general practitioners to use. Although it is possible that you could manage on your own, it will definitely be better to have all the big guns on your side.

Make an appointment to see your doctor as soon as possible. In the Workbook at the back of this book there is an information sheet for your doctor (see page 111), which you should fill in and send when you make your appointment. Meanwhile, keep on logging your scratches as you have been doing for the past week.

Your doctor can help make sure that you have the steroid and emollient creams and ointments that you need. Together you need to assess the treatment you have been using up until now, how you want to adapt it, and any other needs that you have.

You should discuss:
❑ emollients
❑ topical steroids
❑ your mental state.

All these subjects are dealt with in more detail below. Read this chapter through before you talk to your doctor. You might find it helpful to take this book and your completed worksheets with you to your appointment.

Emollients

Emollients are oils, creams and ointments used to moisturize the skin. It is important that you understand exactly how emollients help with dry skin. A common misconception is that they add moisture to the skin. They don't. Instead, they act as a barrier, reducing the amount of body fluid evaporating from the skin's surface. You should think of them as a prevention of dry skin rather than treatment for dry skin. For this reason it is more important to use them frequently than to apply them in large quantities, as frequent applications will renew the insulation against moisture loss. Large irregular applications will not replace moisture that has already been lost and may just make you feel hot, sticky and uncomfortable.

To protect your skin as much as possible you need to use emollients regularly. As a minimum, you need to apply a cream or ointment all over eczematous areas every morning and evening, and use a bath or shower oil every time you wash. If your eczema is severe you will probably need to apply emollients more often, especially to exposed parts. As your skin improves you can reassess your needs and cut down on the applications, but always err on the frequent side. At the beginning of the programme, the more often you apply emollients the better. If your eczema is severe, you can apply emollients every hour and they will still be doing some good. I know it seems disruptive and boring, but it is just the kick-start your skin needs, and it doesn't have to take very long.

Using emollients

Act to prevent dry skin, don't react to dry skin!
Only a shine is required.

Put on emollients
thinly
     gently
          quickly
               frequently.
Don't wake up your skin!

The way you use emollients is important, too. It is all too easy to use the application time to have a good old scratch, and your skin can end up raw, scraped and slimy from being smothered in emollient, with you feeling more stressed than when you started. If you get into the habit of putting on emollients correctly it won't take up much time and will become an automatic, easy and trouble-free exercise. All you need is a thin layer, applied gently and quickly, as often as you can. Use the smallest amount necessary to cover the eczema, just until the skin shines. Wipe or smooth the emollient on, rather than rubbing it in. Try to be very gentle and calm – think of putting on emollient as if you're trying to collect a teddy bear in need of a wash from the arms of a sleeping baby. You don't want to wake your skin up!

Your doctor or pharmacist will probably have suggestions for the right emollients for your skin. As a general guide, if your skin is very dry you may need an ointment, and if it is moderately dry you may need a cream. Ointments act as more effective barriers to moisture loss, which is why they are useful for very dry skins. You may need different emollients for different parts of your body, and special formulations exist for some areas, such as your scalp.

Types of emollients

Creams:
        Thin creams for general use
        Thick creams for special use on driest areas
Ointments
Bath additives
Soap substitutes
Scalp oil or mousse

However, it is important to find the emollient that is right for you. Although my skin was extremely dry I found that ointments felt heavy and uncomfortable, and was happier using creams at a very high application rate. Conversely, a friend of mine with bad eczema had moderately dry skin, but found that ointments were more convenient because he did not have to apply them as often. You also need to take into account any sensitivities; creams are more likely to irritate sensitive skin than ointments.

It is a good idea to decant some emollient from the large tub in which it is supplied into smaller containers to have to hand wherever you need them. How about one in the kitchen (for whenever you dry your hands), one in the living room (to put on while watching television), one in the office and one in the bedroom? There are two reasons for this: you use the emollient more regularly if it is always to hand, and constantly dipping into large containers can turn them into reservoirs for germs.

Wetting your skin washes out oils that naturally protect against moisture loss – this is why it is important to use emollients whenever you wash. Your doctor will be able to recommend a suitable oil to use in the bath or shower. Soap can be very drying, and it is a good idea to use a soap substitute such as aqueous cream instead. Apply it all over before a bath or shower, then wet and gently massage (you will get quite a satisfying lather), and rinse off. You should always apply your usual emollient as soon as you dry off.

Discuss your past experiences with your doctor – together you will be able to identify the best emollients for your needs.

Remember:

Emollients help to reduce symptoms caused by dry skin, including itchiness. They will lessen the discomfort and will help you to scratch less. You should apply them as often as possible: thinly, gently, quickly and frequently.

Topical steroids

Steroids are a relatively recent stage in the treatment of eczema (and many other diseases). The first synthetic steroid was manufactured in the 1950s. Today there are four main groups of steroids, divided according to potency. They all work in the same way, calming down inflammation by blocking the unusual biochemical processes at work in eczematous skin. Appendix 1 (see page 97) shows a list of steroids in the different potency groups.

The word 'topical' is used to describe a medicine that is applied to the skin. Other forms of steroid are oral (given by mouth, mostly as a pill) or intra-muscular (injected into the muscles). Steroids used to treat eczema are usually topical, except when the eczema is very severe.

Doctors and patients alike are concerned about the effects of long-term steroid use. Steroids are powerful medicines, and they can have side-effects, such as thinning of the skin and acne-like rashes. However, remember that side-effects are caused by inappropriate use of steroids. Eczema sufferers, who are often prescribed steroids over long periods of time, frequently become very anxious about side-effects, overlooking the good effects of correct topical steroid therapy. Unfortunately, this can lead to steroids being used incorrectly.

Patients who are worried about the steroids they are using cut down on the amount that is applied, or ask their doctors to prescribe less strong formulations. Doctors themselves are sensibly cautious about topical steroids; they know they can be used inappropriately, with disastrous results. (This is exactly what

happened to me. I asked my doctors to prescribe weaker formulations, and I tried to wean myself off steroids by mixing them
with emollient so that I was applying a diluted dose.) This can
result in inadequate treatment. The weaker dose is relatively in-
effective, and so is used for a longer period of time, sometimes
indefinitely. You can end up using **more steroid** rather than less.

The dermatologists who developed this programme found
that, with Habit Reversal, you can use strong steroids for a much
shorter length of time, and get a much better result. Chronic
eczematous skin will respond quickly to high steroid applications
when all three treatment elements are used simultaneously (emollients, steroids, habit reversal). After the skin has responded the
applications can be stopped. This results in **less steroid** being
used overall.

You probably already know that strong steroids should not be
used on delicate skin, for example, on the face. Your doctor will
prescribe different strengths for different areas of the body, and
you should stick to these.

You will usually be applying the steroids once or twice a day,
according to your doctor's instructions. You should always use
emollients at the same time, applying the emollient *over* the
steroid. Never be tempted to use the steroid cream or ointment
as an emollient. It may help to think of the emollient as the cling
film that you use to cover the skin-and-topical-steroid sandwich
you have made, to keep it fresh.

As well as the potency of the steroid, the time over which it is
applied must be carefully assessed. Eczema sufferers often fear
that steroids are becoming less and less effective. Their skin clears,
but as soon as the steroids are stopped the eczema comes back.
This can be because the steroid is being stopped too soon.

The Look Good Point

When your eczema improves your skin heals in two stages: obvious healing and hidden healing. The first stage is visible; the skin's surface, the epidermis, gradually clears until it reaches a point where it looks completely healthy. We call this the Look Good Point. The second stage is not visible, and people with eczema are often unaware of it. At the Look Good Point, the dermis (the deeper layer of the skin) is still inflamed and eczematous, and during hidden healing the inflammation recedes until the skin is healthy all the way through. If treatment is stopped at the Look Good Point, the eczema can quickly relapse.

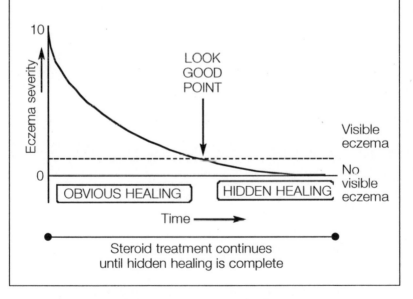

As the eczema begins to clear, the visual impression improves. The skin reaches a point where the surface looks good but the underlying hidden layers are still inflamed. If the steroid is stopped the surface layers will quickly become eczematous again because the skin underneath has never completely healed. Often patients do not have this explained properly to them, and this contributes greatly to the misuse of steroids.

To ensure proper healing with chronic eczema, the full steroid treatment may need to be continued for two weeks after the surface layers look clear (the Look Good Point). This gives the deeper layers time to heal, and ensures that the eczema has completely responded to the treatment.

It sounds like a contradiction, but using stronger steroids for longer in the early stages of treatment will mean that you use fewer steroids overall. I was very nervous about using a strong steroid at the start of the programme, and kept trying to reduce the treatment as soon as my skin looked slightly better. Stick with it, and you will end up with clear skin that stays clear, without steroids.

Remember:

Stronger steroid treatment for a sufficient length of time is more effective than weak steroids continued indefinitely. In chronic eczema, apply Topical steroid to the eczematous skin until the Look Good Point, plus two weeks for hidden healing. The whole process will take perhaps four to six weeks.

Mental state

Do you ever feel like I used to about your skin? Do you find yourself thinking that you had better just get used to the discomfort and misery of eczema, because nothing can be done about it? Do you feel that modern medicine has nothing much to offer you?

This sort of no-hope feeling is very common, both among people with eczema and the people – doctors, family and friends – who care for them. An important part of this programme is to turn around your attitude, so that you are managing your skin rather than being managed by it. You need to shift from a passive to an active frame of mind. You have already started this process by reading this book and beginning the programme.

The doctors who developed this programme realized that the more a patient was involved in the treatment, the better the results. They saw that the more patients knew about the reasons why they had eczema, the better they were able to understand and control it. That is why this book has gone into quite a lot of detail about eczema, dry skin, scratching and Habit Reversal.

Throughout this programme, *you* will be in the driving seat, *not* your skin. If you decide right at the start to stick with all the exercises and treatments, you will feel more and more enabled and in control. Eventually you will realize that this positive attitude, which you work at maintaining now, is there all the time. Don't worry about 'failing' any of the stages, or whether this means that you have blown the whole programme and will never be free of eczema. Some of us find it easy to be defeatist and pessimistic now because we have been disappointed, or set ourselves impossible targets, in the past. Progress is never smooth; we all have our bad days. Don't let a bad day spoil things. Each stage of this programme is well within anyone's abilities as long as they follow the guidelines.

Occasionally people may not be able to get cracking on their own. People who have struggled with eczema for a long time

The Attitude Shift

Chronic eczema		Clear skin
Lack of information	**The Combined**	Get informed
Unhelpful advice	**Approach**	Get cracking
'Learn to live with it'	⟶	Get results
Passive and Pessimistic Attitude		**Active and Optimistic Attitude**

often become quite distraught about their skin. There are all sorts of reactions to prolonged distress of this kind.

My eczema caused a reactive depression that became clinical, taking on a life of its own and becoming an illness in its own right. I needed antidepressants to treat it. I would certainly never have managed to finish the programme without dealing with the depression first.

Eczema sufferers may also have problems with anxiety, insomnia and depression. They may turn to alcohol or drugs for support (see Reggie's Case Study on page 19). Or they may develop phobias about dirt, animals, or crowds of people, although this is not common.

If you are worried about any of these problems, or any others that you feel might be connected to your eczema, you must discuss them with your doctor. This applies even if you think that the problem is insignificant, or is not caused by your eczema. Any obstacle that might stand between you and healthy skin is worthy of consideration. Together you will be able to decide whether you need to pay attention to any aspects of your mental state that might stop you from completing the programme.

You may find it hard and even traumatic to talk about subjects like this. People with eczema often get used to dismissing problems, thinking that they should not make a fuss about things that cannot be helped. So it can be quite stressful to admit to them.

It is tempting to think that as your skin gets better any problems will disappear. And indeed, they might. But on the other hand, they might not. And they might stop your skin from getting better at all.

Remember:

Your doctor is trained to deal with stress-related problems, and will not be shocked by whatever you have to say. He or she also has specially trained colleagues that can be enlisted to help. You need to deal with any problems now, to ensure that you get rid of your eczema and any other conditions that the eczema might have caused.

Levels 1 and 2 Treatment Plan

Chart 5: Levels 1 and 2 Treatment Plan (see page 105), will be a record of what steroids and emollients you and your doctor have decided on. You can either complete it with your doctor or when you get back from your appointment. Make sure you include all the different emollients (cream or ointments for different areas, soap substitutes, bath/shower oils, etc.), and details of when you will use them.

You are likely to have more than one type of steroid, for use on different areas, so record them too. The chart has a form for noting when you have applied the steroid, morning and evening, for two weeks. (Some will be for once a day only – you choose when.) Fill this in every time you apply them; it will help to re-inforce the treatment plan.

The temptation will be to cut down on applications as your skin gets better, but do stick with the schedule, for all the reasons covered in this chapter. As your eczema improves, you and your doctor will be able to adapt your treatments correspondingly, and draw up a new version of the chart.

NEXT APPOINTMENT

Your next appointment with your doctor should be in about four to six weeks, to admire your progress and review your emollient and steroid requirements. However, do go back straight away if anything unusual happens, for example, if your skin gets infected or you suspect a new emollient is not suit-ing you.

Please do not go on to the next chapter until you have been to your doctor and planned your Levels 1 and 2 treatments.

Points to remember

1   You will need your doctor's support throughout the programme. Make an appointment and send off the letter on page 111 as soon as possible.

2   Emollients help to reduce symptoms caused by dry skin, including itchiness. They will lessen the discomfort, and will help you to scratch less. You should apply them as often as you can: thinly, gently, quickly and frequently.

3   Stronger steroid treatment for sufficient length of time is more effective than weak steroids continued in-definitely. Apply to the eczematous skin until the Look Good Point, plus two weeks for hidden healing.

4 Discuss any other problems (even those that you think are unimportant or not related to your eczema) with your doctor. Problems that are not dealt with now might prevent you from finishing this programme.

'The worst thing about having bad eczema was the personal hygiene side,' says Laura. 'People look at you and think you're disgusting.' Laura, now 34, hasn't had a problem with her skin since completing the programme six years ago. 'My skin used to feel so tight across my back that I felt I would crack if I leant forward.' Laura had eczema as a baby, which became very severe throughout her teens, until her skin was inflamed from top to toe. Her wrists became so badly damaged that burns dressings were used to protect them. Several hospitalizations and a very restricted diet bought only limited relief, until she was referred to Chelsea and Westminster Hospital after moving to London. Now, she looks back on having severe eczema and says, 'I can hardly believe that was me. Now I can eat what I want, go swimming; I can wear what I choose and people don't look at me with revulsion. It feels like another life.'

chapter five

HABIT REVERSAL: ADDRESSING THE PROBLEM

You're always being told 'don't scratch', 'don't scratch' and having your hands slapped, so you do it furtively, you can't stop even when somebody is taking your picture.

You have been to see your doctor and are armed with emollients, steroids, an application plan, and everything else that you need. Now you are ready to begin the next step of the programme. This is where the fun starts!

We have established that your eczema will never clear while you are still scratching, and you have monitored your scratching for a week to understand how much, when, why and where you do it. Next we are going to develop an action plan to replace the scratching with healing, without battles of will that are impossible to win. You are going to re-learn your response, not only to itching, but also to the other things that make you scratch. At the end of this process you won't be automatically scratching all the time, and you won't have to struggle not to.

Choose a time when you will not be interrupted for an hour or so to read and practise the exercises in this chapter.

ABC of scratching

Let's have a look at what happens when you scratch. The scratching episode really starts *before* you actually scratch, when you experience the impulse to scratch. This antecedent was originally an itch, but may now be a variety of other feelings or situations as well. The impulse stimulates a particular behaviour: scratching. The final part of the scratching episode is what happens afterwards: the physical, emotional and social consequences. These include the physical damage that scratching does to your skin; the distress, relief and guilt that you may feel emotionally; and the (usually negative) reactions of others.

This sequence can be summarized as three steps: Antecedent; Behaviour; Consequence. The aim of Habit Reversal is to replace this undesirable sequence with a new, desirable one. In the desirable sequence, scratching as a response to the impulse is replaced with a new, non-damaging behaviour. The new response is introduced immediately following the impulse, like night follows day. This becomes the new habit. The final consequence, rather than damage, is healing. This follows inevitably, when the behaviour changes. Sounds good, eh?

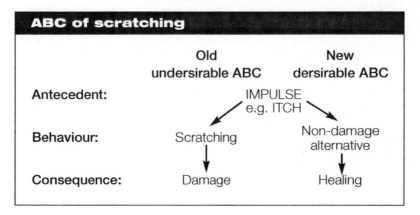

ABC of scratching		
	Old undersirable ABC	New dersirable ABC
Antecedent:	IMPULSE e.g. ITCH	
Behaviour:	Scratching	Non-damage alternative
Consequence:	Damage	Healing

Switching from scratching

So, what is this alternative, non-damaging behaviour? First, let's look at the behaviour we want to replace. Scratching can be divided into two stages:

Stage A: going to the area to be scratched
Stage B: scratching the area.

We need to replace both stages, and the new replacement behaviour has to be something that will rule out doing the old behaviour at the same time.

Stage A of the new behaviour is clenching your fists gently for a count of 30 seconds, with the arms held comfortably at the sides of the body.

Stage B of the new behaviour is gently pinching or pressing a nail onto the area of skin that would have been scratched, until the impulse to scratch has gone.*

Have a couple of practice runs. You feel an itch, say, on your knee (for the rehearsal, imagine this if necessary). Instead of automatically moving your hand towards your knee, you clench both fists at your sides for a slow count of 30. Fix your thoughts on something calm and pleasant while you count. Then, if your knee is still itching, gently pinch or press a nail into the itchy area. Don't move, just maintain a gentle pressure until the itch subsides. Easy, wasn't it?

---

* It always goes ... but it does come back again, at least to begin with, so go back to Stage A!

Try it again, with an itch on your elbow. *Fists ... count ... something nice ... press.* Now, how about one on your forehead?

You don't need to be particularly fierce about clenching your fists unless you find that it helps. Do avoid putting all the frustration of the itch into a really hard fist squeeze because that will destroy the action's calming, non-aggressive feeling, and simply work you up to have a really good go at the itch when your concentration wavers. Likewise, at Stage B, don't let the press or pinch turn into a rub, or even the tiniest scratch. Just a gentle clench is totally effective, but it's just not what you are used to. Quite often, by the time you get to the end of the 30 seconds the impulse will have gone, and there will be no need to go on to the press/pinch stage.

The new behaviour has been designed to address both the specific, itch-related scratching and the generalized habit scratching that we know characterizes chronic eczema. Stage A counters the habit scratching. Stage B counters the itch-scratching.

Practise the two-stage sequence several times a day for the next few days, just as you have done for the examples above. You need to get this set of reactions into your subconscious. That way, it becomes your new, healing habit.

From now on do it for real, too. Every time you are aware of an impulse to scratch, whether it is an itch or because of something else, clench your fists for 30 seconds and then press the area you would have scratched if you still need to. If you have already started scratching, which will probably happen at first, go into the sequence as soon as you realize. Your trained team of 'click'-ers can continue to help, either by saying 'click!' or waving a friendly fist if they see you scratching, which will remind you to clench your fists and count to 30.

You should still carry on logging the times when you actually do scratch (or rub, or pick) as before. You should not log the times when you carry out the new behaviour instead of scratching. Just click when you actually have scratched. *Chart 6: Habit Reversal* (see page 107) includes a table for registering your scratching over the next few weeks. As the number comes down you will be rewarded by your skin healing.

Don't worry if all this sounds as if it will take up a lot of your time. Just think of all the scratching episodes that last for much longer than 30 seconds. Some of them last for several minutes, especially if you count the Consequences stage of feeling bad and having to go and put on cream or washing the area you have just marmalized. You will end up by saving all that time.

Remember:

You need to replace your old scratching with a new behaviour. Stage A is clenching your fists for a count of 30 seconds. Stage B is gently pinching or pressing the area until the impulse to scratch has gone.

Practise your new behaviour several times a day for the first few days. *Fists ... count ... something nice ... press.* The good news is that if, at the end of the 30 seconds clenching, there is no more impulse to scratch, you **do not** need to go on to the skin pinch/press stage.

From now on, start replacing all your scratching with the new behaviour.

Danger times

There will be some situations when the new behaviour is impractical, or the impulse to scratch is either very strong or very common. Have a look at the most scratchy times on your completed *Chart 1: Registration*. There will be some that occur frequently, possibly several times every day. These are the times when you are most likely to go back to the old behaviour of scratching and damaging. You need reinforcements for these danger times.

Firstly, it might be possible to avoid some of the difficult situations altogether, at least for the next three or four weeks. Can you get someone else to mow the lawn/organize the event/do the supermarket shopping/wash the dishes? Can you put off redecorating the spare room or confronting the difficult person – or whatever it is that provokes your scratching? If you can dispense with some of the danger times, even if only temporarily, you will significantly cut down on the amount you scratch.

Many of the scratchy situations will not be possible to avoid, and for these you can have an alternative action plan. You need to adapt each of the indispensable situations so that they are no longer danger times. There are three main tactics for getting through these situations without scratching:

❏ plan ahead
❏ do it quickly
❏ keep your hands busy.

For example, two of my most scratch-prone situations were getting up in the morning and going to bed at night. These are very common danger times. The solution for me was to plan ahead, and lay out the emollients that I needed to apply and the clothes I would wear before I did anything else. Then I would have a shower, dry off, put on emollients and get dressed as one quick operation, rather than wander around scratching while I looked for items of clothing and tubes of cream. I needed to concentrate at first, but it worked. I carried out the same sequence for going to bed.

Keeping your hands busy is a very important tactic, especially for the relatively passive situations like talking on the telephone, reading or watching television. In these situations it is easy to scratch distractedly for hours on end. Try keeping a doodle pad by the phone, and put a sign on the wall saying 'PICK UP THE BIRO' where you will see it as soon as you reach for the receiver. If you are right-handed always pick up the phone with your left hand. If one hand is holding the receiver and the other is doodling you can't scratch.

Some people have had very good results from taking up a manual activity such as knitting while watching television. Other options include putting signs up to remind yourself not to scratch in places like the bathroom or toilet, developing rituals such as patting rather than rubbing dry after showers or baths, and getting up for ten minutes when scratching in bed. Bed is for sleeping, not scratching!

A simple technique that I relied on for a wide range of situations was to do everything with two hands. Many of my danger times were when carrying out an activity that I did not like and which brought on mild stress, such as housework, driving in heavy traffic, or looking for things. I tended to do the job with one hand, the other being permanently engaged in scratching my back, hip, neck or forehead. Switching to holding the vacuum cleaner, car steering wheel, or file I was carrying with both hands prevented scratching immediately. You could put 'BOTH HANDS' signs up at critical places around the house or office if you think this would help.

Sometimes, all your best-laid plans will fall apart and you will just have to have a really good old scratch. If this happens, don't beat yourself up. We're all human. But don't use it as an excuse to wreck your record for the rest of the day, either. It's surprisingly tempting to look for reasons to let yourself off the hook – a bit like carrying on bingeing all day after you've broken your diet with a chocolate biscuit. Or you might feel that you've failed and there's no point in trying. Neither of these is the right reaction. Just forgive yourself, and move on. Carry on with the good work as soon as you can.

Self-prescription

On a spare piece of paper, write down some ideas for adapting your first difficult situation. These need not be taken from the examples above; the only requirement is that you are unable to scratch while doing them. Try to involve the three tactics: planning ahead, doing it quickly, and keeping your hands busy.

From the list of ideas you have jotted down, choose the one or two that will work best for you, the simpler the better. The easier they are to remember and carry out, the more likely you are to make a success of them. **This is your self-prescription for this situation, the treatment you prescribe yourself to control the danger time.**

Repeat the exercise for your other difficult situations, until you have a self-prescription for each one. Then enter these on *Chart 6: Habit Reversal.* If you find that the theory does not work so well in practice you can always come back and refine them.

Chart 6 - example

Otherwise – Self-prescription:

1 **Getting up:** lay out all clothes and emollients beforehand, dress and leave the room quickly.

2 **On the telephone:** at home, use a doodle pad. At work, play with an executive desk toy, doodle or take notes. Have a pad, pen, toy and reminder sign beside all phones.

3 **Driving:** always have music on and tap along to it on the steering wheel with both hands. Keep a selection of tapes in the car for when the radio is too annoying, and a 'BOTH HANDS' sign on the dashboard.

4 **Before difficult social occasions:** deep yoga breathing for two minutes, practise new behaviour five times in a row, tell myself that everything will be fine and even if it isn't, it won't matter and I won't want to scratch.

Remember:

Use your self-prescription to replace scratching in difficult situations where the new behaviour needs some back-up. Plan ahead; do it quickly; keep your hands busy.

What now?

Over the next two weeks, starting right now, you will be doing three things:

1 Level 1 and 2 Treatment as discussed with your doctor, according to the principles in Chapter 4. Follow the Levels 1 and 2 Treatment Plan.

2 Start Level 3: introducing the new behaviour to replace the old scratching, and using your self-prescription behaviour for difficult situations. Remember, you need all three levels to heal chronic eczema.

3 Carrying on registering your ever-decreasing scratching on *Chart 6: Habit Reversal.*

I suggest that you re-read this chapter after one week, just to refresh your memory of all the new techniques you have learned, and to trigger any better theories on how to manage difficult situations.

Good luck!

See you in two weeks.

Points to remember

1 You need to replace your old scratching with a new behaviour. Stage A is clenching your fists for a count of 30 seconds. Stage B is gently pinching or pressing the area until the impulse to scratch has gone.

2 Practise your new behaviour several times a day for the first few days. *Fists ... count ... something nice ... press.*

3 From now on start replacing all your scratching with the new behaviour. If at the end of A the impulse has gone, there is no need for B.

4 Use your self-prescription to prevent scratching in difficult situations where the new behaviour needs some backup. Plan ahead; do it quickly; keep your hands busy.

5 All three levels of treatment are needed to heal chronic atopic eczema.

chapter six

HABIT REVERSAL: BEATING THE PROBLEM

My clothes used to stick to the weeping scratches – I remember having to rip tights off.

Welcome back, and I hope you have had a productive two weeks. If all has gone well you will have accomplished a lot. You have:

- ❏ Started a new application plan for Levels 1 and 2 (dry skin and eczema);
- ❏ Learnt a new ABC behaviour sequence to replace the bad old scratching ABC;
- ❏ Started to replace your scratching with the new behaviour;
- ❏ Developed self-prescriptions for difficult situations;
- ❏ Carried on registering your scratches on a daily basis.

Choose a quiet hour to read this chapter and complete the exercises. Let's start with a review of your progress. Get out *Chart 3: Eczema Review* and *Chart 6: Habit Reversal*.

Eczema severity and distribution

How bad is your eczema now, on the 0–10 scale? The combination of Level 1 and 2 Treatment, and the beginning of Habit Reversal, is likely to have had quite an effect on the severity of your eczema. Give your eczema a score and enter it into the next column in *Chart 3*.

Where is the eczema worst? Where is the rest? Note it down on *Chart 3*. Compare your eczema now to how it was two weeks ago. Has the distribution changed? Do some areas seem to be improving more quickly than others or is the distribution the same? Fill in a new body map, showing how your eczema is now, and keep it with the first one.

Think about the amounts of old and new eczema that you have, and enter your percentage of old eczema in *Chart 3*. Often the Level 2 Treatment for eczema and itch, appropriate steroid application, will have a very rapid impact on acute eczema. The Habit Reversal is the Level 3 Treatment for scratching, essential for healing chronic eczema. You are using both treatments. Are they both working at the same rate? Has the percentage of old eczema changed compared with two weeks ago? Has anything happened in the past two weeks to cause a flare-up of acute eczema? (We will look at how to deal with flare-ups later.)

Levels 1 and 2 Treatment review

Now, let's think about your treatments. We will look at the Level 3 Treatment, Habit Reversal, in detail later, but it is important to keep reviewing all aspects of your treatment. This is how the Combined Approach works: all the levels have to be addressed together.

LEVEL 1: EMOLLIENTS

How often are you applying the different kinds of emollients? Are you managing to keep to the treatment plan you developed in *Chart 5*? Ask yourself: 'When am I using emollients?' If the answer is 'when my skin is dry' you may have missed the point – you need to *anticipate* drying, and *prevent* it with an emollient application. If you have stepped up the frequency of application (rather than the amount applied at one time), have you noticed your skin becoming less dry? If you have, this is good news, but don't cut down on the applications just yet. Let your skin enjoy being pampered – it deserves it!

LEVEL 2: STEROIDS

Now let's look at steroids. Have you kept up with the treatment plan for the different steroid preparations? Are you happy about the amount you are using? Remember, strong steroid treatment for an appropriate length of time is more effective than a weaker dose used indefinitely, so don't worry if it seems you are using a lot of steroid at the moment. Your skin needs the anti-inflammatory action of the steroid. Remember hidden healing: you need to apply the steroid for two weeks after the Look Good Point to enable the skin to heal completely. If you stop the steroid too early the eczema will relapse.

You might find it helpful to go back and re-read the Emollients and Steroid sections of Chapter 4 at this stage, just to review the principles of Levels 1 and 2 Treatment.

Remember:

Stick to your treatment plan for emollients and steroids, even if your skin is getting much better. Give time for hidden healing.

The Combined Approach works by addressing all three levels of eczema together.

Level 3 Treatment: Habit Reversal

SCRATCHING FREQUENCY AND CAUSE

How has your scratching frequency, recorded on *Chart 6*, changed? Are you still scratching as often as you were at the beginning of the two weeks, or do the numbers decrease? If you are managing to carry out the new anti-scratching behaviour you learned two weeks ago, the scratching frequency will have started to go down.

What about the way you are scratching? Think back over the times when you have scratched during the last two weeks (unless you are a genius who never scratched again from the day you learnt the new behaviour!). Has your technique changed? You might find that the scratching is getting less intense, because they are just little distracted scratches before you realize what you are doing and clench your fists. Or you might find that the scratches are more intense, because you have decreased the amount of habit scratching you are doing, but still find that you are responding aggressively to particular situations or itches. In this case, you might want to review your self-prescription for those situations.

What percentage of your scratching is coming from itch now? This may have changed from two weeks ago, depending on how your particular pattern of Habit Reversal is developing. Are you avoiding habit scratching more and therefore is more of your scratching in response to an itch? Or are you using the new behaviour of pinching or pressing to avoid scratching itches, so that more of your scratching is coming from habit? Enter a percentage of scratching coming from itch in *Chart 6*.

Remember:

Keep replacing scratching with your new behaviour, and use self-prescriptions for especially scratchy situations. Plan ahead; do it quickly; keep your hands busy.

TROUBLESHOOTING

What if your scratching frequency has not fallen? Hopefully, this will not be the case, but if it is, think about the new behaviour. Are you having trouble remembering to do it? Do you really understand what to do? If you are not sure, try re-reading Chapter 5, and then write out what to do in your own words, covering:

1 The ABC sequence of scratching (antecedent, behaviour, consequence);
2 The way you want to change to a new sequence which does not involve scratching;
3 The two stages of scratching (moving your hand to the area and scratching the area);
4 The two new stages that you want to replace the scratching (clenching fists and pressing);
5 Self-prescriptions for difficult situations.

This is a good way of making sure you understand every step. Another way is to explain the programme to someone else. If this helps, and you think that you now understand something that you were not sure of before, then go back and do another week of new behaviour and monitoring, and then come back to this chapter.

You will find Habit Reversal much easier if you are getting all the benefits from Levels 1 and 2 Treatment. Make sure you are sticking scrupulously to your emollients and steroids, plus any other treatments your doctor may have prescribed for you. If it seems hard going, just remember that it can only get easier, and one day soon you'll have smooth, clear, comfortable skin and all the battles will have been worth it.

Focus times

Now that your scratching frequency is decreasing and you have put special behaviours into place for difficult situations, you may notice a pattern in the distribution of your scratching over a 24-hour period. When do most of the difficult situations occur? At the start of the day, at lunchtime, mid-afternoon, early evening, late evening, middle of the night? Think about when you still scratch most.

Quite often, people find that scratching times get localized as the overall levels go down. You take away the constant background scratching and are left with the particularly scratchy situations. This means that, as you break the habit of continual scratching, you have to work less hard on anti-scratching behaviour through most of the day. This frees you up to concentrate on the most risky times.

There are some particularly common times for high scratching risk. Many people encounter a lot of their difficult situations when they are getting up in the morning, when they come home and unwind at the end of the day, and when they are tired or going to bed last thing at night. Think about your pattern of risky times. You may not have this same pattern, especially if you do shift work or are at home during the day, but you are likely to be able to identify two or three time slots when you do most of your scratching.

Behavioural change is more successful when you can focus your attention and get positive results. By now you may only need to focus on, say, three hours in each 24. This will seem a much more manageable task for the next two weeks. Using these times as focus times, when you concentrate your anti-scratching behaviour, will seem like a much easier approach than having to concentrate all the time.

Some focus times will involve several situations when you are likely to scratch, and you might find it is useful to put together a little routine, which you use to get through them in one piece. The routine will really be a sequence of self-prescriptions, for each individual danger situation that makes up the focus time. You may have to devise some new ones if thinking about focus times has brought some new scratchy situations to your attention.

A common focus time is just after coming home at the end of the day. This is an unwinding time, when you may be feeling rather tired and let your vigilance drop. You may need to change out of outdoor or work clothes, and put on emollients, and often this becomes an occasion for a routine scratching session. I used to find I couldn't relax easily until I had gone upstairs and spent a good 45 minutes inspecting my skin: picking; scratching; putting on cream; and finally dressing in casual clothes and coming back down again. It fulfilled the same psychological need as coming home and having a cup of tea. An alternative routine for this focus time could be to jump straight into the shower, so that your skin feels clean with no tempting bits to pick at, apply emollients, dress, put the kettle on and then sit down with a paper or book for ten minutes.

Complete *Chart 7: Focus times for anti-scratching behaviour* (see page 110), shading in the times when you will concentrate your efforts. When you have shaded in your focus times, fill in the table with your self-prescriptions for each one. This will help you to concentrate on what to do to make your focus times really effective, and it will make shifting the last bit of chronic eczema a lot easier. See below for typical afternoon focus times.

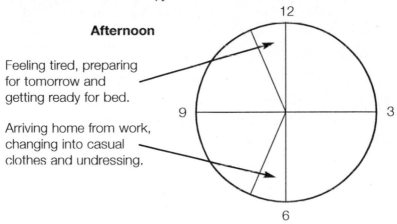

Afternoon

Feeling tired, preparing for tomorrow and getting ready for bed.

Arriving home from work, changing into casual clothes and undressing.

Times	Circumstances	Self-prescription
4 **11:00 to 12:00 pm**	Feeling tired, preparing for tomorrow and getting ready for bed.	Bedtime at 11:00pm — before I get too tired. Develop a going-to-bed routine: tomorrow's clothes (if getting up is a focus time); wash & clean teeth; emollients & steroids; straight to bed; listen to relaxation tape or read for 10 minutes.

Remember:

Be prepared for focus times. It will be much easier to concentrate on your self-prescriptions and new behaviour for just a few hours in a day than for the whole twenty-four.

What now?

Over the next two weeks, carry on replacing your scratching with the new behaviour as before. Use the focus times you have identified to concentrate on the scratchiest periods of the day. During focus times, use self-prescriptions to avoid scratching, and the replacement behaviour (*Fists ... count ... something nice ... press)* if you do feel the urge to scratch. Keep logging and recording any scratching that is still happening on a copy of *Chart 6*; it is important to stay aware of your progress. I suggest you re-read this chapter after one week, just to remind yourself of the concept of focus times.

Have a focused two weeks!

Points to remember

1 Stick to your treatment plan for emollients and steroids, even if your skin is getting much better. Give time for hidden healing. The Combined Approach works by addressing all three levels of eczema together.

2 Keep replacing scratching with your new behaviour, and use self-prescriptions for especially scratchy situations. Plan ahead; do it quickly; keep your hands busy.

3 Be prepared for focus times. It will be much easier to concentrate on your self-prescriptions and new behaviour for just a few hours in a day than for the whole twenty-four.

CASE STUDY

Fiona has had bad eczema ever since the age of five, when it flared up on starting junior school. As a little girl, she remembers having to wear bandages around her wrists, elbows and knees, clashing with the pretty dresses she wanted to wear. Now 28, she has just finished the Habit Reversal programme. Previously, Fiona had tried several complementary therapies without success, including homeopathy, Chinese herbs and an exclusion diet, and was amazed by how simple and effective the programme was. 'I cannot believe, after all those years, that there is something that actually works'. She tried Habit Reversal after her psychiatrist brother heard about the programme from doctor friends. It was not a moment too soon. 'I had reached the end of my tether' she remembers. 'I had had four lots of antibiotics in 10 weeks. My skin was constantly infected, red and raw.' Fiona was shocked by her scratching tallies at the start of the course, but they quickly came under control, dropping from 360 scratches a day to just 60 in the first week. She is delighted by the results, and relishing the thought of being able to wear buy short-sleeved tops for the first time in years. 'It's like having completely new skin – it changes your life.'

chapter seven
THE HEALING CURVE

Six years after completing the habit reversal programme, I look at photos and think 'Was that me?' It seems like a different life.

Welcome back again, and I hope you've enjoyed the feeling of regaining more and more control over your skin during focus times! All being well, you'll have:

- ❏ Continued to reinforce the replacement behaviour instead of scratching;
- ❏ Identified two to four focus times during the day when you are most inclined to scratch;
- ❏ Concentrated your replacement behaviour and self-prescriptions on the focus times.

You should be seeing a real improvement in the condition of your skin, and your scratching totals should have fallen considerably. You have every right to feel proud of yourself!

As before, let's start by reviewing your progress over the last two weeks. You will need the charts from the Workbook, and a quiet hour when you will not be disturbed.

Eczema severity and distribution

Fill in the next column on *Chart 3*, giving your eczema an overall score from 0 to 10. How has this changed from two weeks ago?

Think about the balance of chronic and acute eczema, and enter a score for percentage old eczema. Is the score now different from the previous entries? Can you explain why it is or is not different? Remember, acute eczema responds to Levels 1 and 2 treatments (emollients and steroids) while chronic eczema needs all three levels of treatment, including Habit Reversal. You have been using both for the last four or five weeks. The acute eczema will clear quickly with the right treatment, but can flare up again for a few days at a time. The chronic eczema will clear more slowly, but once cleared it will not return unless scratching resumes.

Think about the pattern of eczema distribution as well. By now you may be finding that most of your skin is clearing apart from one or two stubborn spots. Or it may all be clearing at the same rate, with no particular problem areas. Note down the pattern of your eczema on *Chart 3*. It might be easier to see which areas are clearing fastest and which ones need a little extra attention if you shade in another body map and compare it with the first two. If you have stubborn areas of chronic eczema (and most people will have), think about when you scratch them. Can you improve on your self-prescriptions for these areas?

Levels 1 and 2 Treatment review

As always, we need to remember that all three levels of treatment must work together to treat chronic eczema successfully.

LEVEL 1: EMOLLIENTS

By now you should be used to applying emollients regularly, before your skin feels dry. You may even be finding that you can apply them less often and still not experience dry skin. This is fine, but be vigilant and ready to increase the frequency at the slightest sign that your skin would like to be coddled. Emollients are still your easiest and most basic maintenance technique.

Remember:

Apply emollients little, often and gently.

LEVEL 2: STEROIDS

If you had any areas of eczema that had reached the Look Good Point two weeks ago, they will now have come to the end of the two-week hidden healing period, and you can stop applying steroids to them. Other areas will probably still be clearing, and you should keep up the applications according to your treatment plan. Look at your skin when you apply your steroids, and make sure you know which patches are clearing, which are being stubborn, and which have cleared but are in the hidden healing period. This may sound unnecessary, but it is surprisingly easy to get into a routine of using treatments without taking much notice of the exact state of the skin you are applying them to, especially if you are deliberately applying them quickly and efficiently as part of a self-prescription. Keep track of the healing stage that each patch of eczema has reached.

Remember:

Stick to your treatment plan for emollients and steroids, even if your skin is getting much better. Give time for hidden healing.

The Combined Approach works by addressing all three levels of eczema together.

Level 3 Treatment: Habit Reversal

Looking at *Chart 6*, how has your scratching frequency changed? What is the balance between habit scratching and scratching in response to an itch? Enter a score for percentage of scratching coming from an itch. Think about the reasons for your answer. Are you doing better at preventing habit scratching or itch-response scratching with your replacement behaviour? How far are you on the way to getting rid of both?

It might help to remember that itching is the feeling of healing: skin on the mend will itch as the inflammation goes down and normal structure is rebuilt. Itching is a good sign – as long as further damage is avoided. You might be finding that your scratching is falling more and more into the focus times you identified two weeks ago, as the background levels continue to fall. Carry on using self-prescriptions and concentrate your efforts on these times. Gradually, you will get out of the habit of scratching even in these more difficult situations, and your scratching will decrease down to background levels, which are, of course, themselves decreasing down to nothing. You should ultimately be aiming for fewer than ten episodes per day (five is possible).

Remember:

Itching is the feeling of healing. Carry on doing Habit Reversal, concentrating especially on focus times, until you eliminate habit scratching and itch-response scratching. Aim for fewer than ten episodes per day.

The healing curve

Are you bracing yourself to learn yet another set of exercises and new behaviours? Well, relax – you've done most of the hard work. You now know the techniques: scratching registration; replacement behaviour; self-prescriptions; and focus times. This is the end of the learning part of the programme. Now all you have to do is keep vigilant!

Everyone will have a different rate of healing. You may already have daily scratch totals in single figures, and the majority of your skin at or near the Look Good Point. Or you may still be working towards this. All you have to do is keep on sliding down the healing curve, using all the tools that the Combined Approach has given you.

The healing curve is an imaginary graph of the severity of your eczema over time. It is at a high level when you start the programme, and decreases as you go through each stage until it gets down to nothing: clear skin. After four weeks of the Combined Approach, using Habit Reversal as well as steroids and emollients at the right levels, you should be well on your way down the healing curve. It is important to understand how each of the treatment levels should be handled as your skin gets better. You don't, after all, want to be doing all three forever. The key to knowing when to stop a treatment is this: **stop when your skin no longer needs the treatment.**

When you combine moisturizers and topical steroids with stopping scratching your chronic eczema will clear up, because there is nothing to keep it there. When this happens, and your skin reaches the Look Good Point, you can stop your Habit Reversal because it has done its job. In practice you will stop naturally, because as you lose the habit of scratching you will no

DISCONTINUING TREATMENT LEVELS

Each treatment is stopped when the skin no longer needs it: Habit Reversal when scratching has stopped and the skin reaches the Look Good Point; steroid treatment when hidden healing is complete; emollients may continue to be applied at a lower frequency for a longer time.

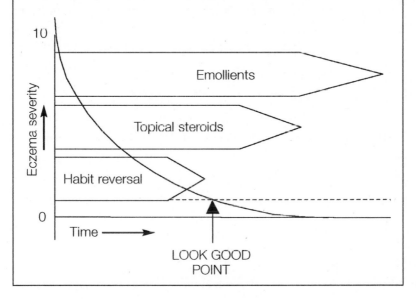

longer need to do the replacement behaviour. It probably is not a good idea to decide 'right, no need to try not to scratch anymore' – this could lead to the subconscious attitude that it's OK to scratch, now that your skin is clear. Of course, if you do this chronic eczema can return.

The next stage is to stop the steroid applications. Again, this only happens when your skin no longer needs them, i.e. at the end of the hidden healing period, two weeks after the Look Good Point. Stopping the steroids before this just allows the eczema to flare up again. After hidden healing, the skin is no longer inflamed and so doesn't need the anti-inflammatory action of the steroid. Now it is safe to stop Level 2 Treatment.

This only leaves Level 1 Treatment: emollients. As your skin gets better it regains its natural waterproof and elastic qualities, and the need to apply emollients several times a day decreases. You have probably already found that the amount of emollient you need has gone down from the very high levels at the beginning of the programme. But do take care. Letting your skin dry out is one of the quickest ways to start the whole dryness – itchiness – inflammation – scratching – eczema cycle off all over again. More than this, regularly moisturizing your skin will allow it to get better faster than it otherwise would. You may never want to stop using emollients altogether. The trick will be to adapt them to the best long-term maintenance plan that fits in with your lifestyle and keeps your skin in top condition.

Remember:

Each treatment is only stopped when the skin no longer needs it: Habit Reversal when scratching has stopped (at the Look Good Point); steroid treatment when hidden healing is complete; emollients may continue to be applied at a lower frequency.

Relapse recognition

As you progress down the healing curve, it is quite likely that you will experience some blips of acute eczema. These need to be controlled immediately – you don't want anything to interrupt you on your way to clear skin. As you are atopic you will always be prone to flare-ups, when your skin is irritated or you are stressed or unwell, or in an environment that doesn't suit you. However, with the right management, these relapses can be neutralized as soon as they start and will not become serious. Over time, as your skin gets stronger and more stable, they will become less frequent, and you will be able to stop them before they damage your lovely healthy skin. The trick is to recognize the signs, and start treating them straight away.

There are two sets of signs to look out for in relapse recognition: dryness and roughness, which are treated with emollient therapy; and redness and itchiness, which are treated with topical steroids. Don't worry if you have got past the hidden healing stage and stopped your steroid treatment plan. It is not a step backwards to start using steroids again to treat relapses – in fact it still means you will use less steroid in the long run, because untreated relapses could turn back into chronic eczema, which would require longer-term steroid use.

Treating a relapse is not the same as the longer-term treatment you have been going through for this programme, even though you use the same medicines. A relapse is acute eczema, which we know can appear and vanish within a couple of days. It will only become serious if it is allowed to progress to chronic eczema. If acute treatment is applied early and correctly, within hours, itch is eliminated and scratching need never become established as a habit again. All you have to do is use Level 1 and 2 Treatments to get rid of it as quickly as possible. If you do feel the urge to scratch, get stuck in with the replacement behaviour before you can start scratching!

The doctors who developed this programme found that a standard approach worked well to control relapses. This is what you do:

Sign	Treatment	Duration
Dryness and roughness	Emollients	Increased frequency until dryness goes.
Redness and itchiness (depending on the steroids you have been prescribed; see Appendix 1 for potencies).	Old topical steroids (usually applied twice a day)	Twice a day for 3 days, then once a day for 3 days, then stop!
	New topical steroids (usually applied once a day)	Once a day for 3 days, alternate days for 4 days, then stop!

Following this standard approach means that all acute eczema blips are treated right at the start, when the skin just looks a little dry or red. The standard approach includes three days of obvious and three days of hidden healing. You won't need to carry on applying steroids for the whole two weeks needed when treating chronic eczema. This is because the inflammation in acute eczema can be 'turned off' more quickly. If you catch the blip early you will usually reach the Look Good Point in the first couple of days.

If you get into the habit of noticing your skin every day, for example as part of your continuing emollient applications, you will always be in a position to stop blips in their tracks. They will be a mild inconvenience rather than a major disaster, and will only last for a matter of days, rather than heralding weeks or months of misery.

It is worth thinking about the factors that are likely to lead to a relapse. These generally fall into two categories: unavoidable and avoidable. The main unavoidable factor is atopy, which you can't get rid of. There may be other factors that are always present too, such as an allergy or sensitivity to something that it is hard to avoid, reactions to seasons and climate, or illness. The avoidable factors vary from person to person, and include a wide range of things such as general health, allergies and irritants, exhaustion and stress. Obviously, to get the best from your skin you need to avoid these factors as much as possible, or plan for them in advance. For example, if you know your skin is worse in winter, step up emollient application frequencies and be extra-vigilant for redness and itchiness all through the cold months.

Remember:

Catch acute eczema relapses early. Treat dryness and roughness with extra emollient applications. Treat redness and itchiness with the topical steroid twice a day for three days, then once a day for three days, then stop.

STRESS

One of the most common causes of relapse is stress. You may be finding that as your skin gets better your ability to cope with stress improves. Mine certainly did – situations that would have had me in tears and scratching down to the bone now only provoke a whinging session on the phone to a friend. However, if stress has been a cause of bad flare-ups in the past, you might want to think about being proactive in managing it.

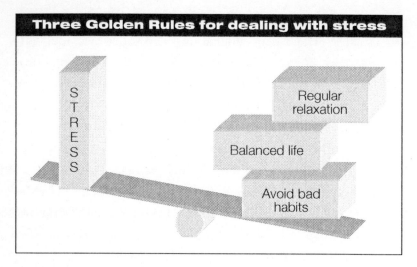

Three Golden Rules for dealing with stress

STRESS

Regular relaxation

Balanced life

Avoid bad habits

There are three golden rules for dealing with stress:

1 Regular relaxation
2 Balance your life
3 Avoid bad habits.

Relaxation can include exercise, and in fact it is common for people to feel less tired and emotional if they take regular exercise and raise their fitness levels. One of the perks of having clear skin is that exercise becomes a pleasure rather than a pain, so this could be a good area to explore. And physical activity can be a terrific outlet for stress. But if you are not fond of physical exercise, any favourite technique, practised frequently, will have a beneficial effect on your stress levels. This could include yoga, meditation, relaxation tapes, music, or just settling down for a private time with a good book. The key is to relax regularly, and not just when you are already feeling frazzled.

Balancing your life involves making sure that each area within your life has enough emphasis. Think about how much time you

The Serenity Prayer

God grant me the serenity
To accept the things I cannot change
The courage to change the things I can
And the wisdom to know the difference

Prayer of St Francis of Assisi

spend working, at home, with friends and on hobbies. It is also important to recognize limits, asking for help if you need it, and if you get sick, not carrying on as if you are well. We all need to learn to accept what we cannot change, and to distinguish things which we can do from impossible tasks. A very easy stress relief technique is to agree with someone: avoid unnecessary confrontations.

Bad habits are easy to fall into, as an escape from stress. These can include abusing caffeine (in tea and coffee), tobacco, alcohol, tranquillizers and sleeping pills. All of these, in the wrong quantities, can raise your stress levels and damage your health. Other important areas are making sure you eat a healthy diet – you don't have to be a nutritionist to ensure you eat plenty of fresh fruit and vegetables, fibre, and high-quality protein and carbohydrates, or a complete idler to ensure you get a good night's sleep. Know when you are tired and do something about it.

If you think that stress management might be a problem for you, then you will almost certainly benefit from taking a more proactive approach. Get a book on stress management, enrol in a relaxation class, join a gym, or talk to your doctor, who will be able to advise you on the best ways to control your stress levels. Nobody can eliminate stress entirely from life. But after all the work you have put in, it would be a shame to let it become a regular cause of acute eczema relapses. I bet there are other areas in your life that could benefit from a little less stress, too!

Remember:

Stress is a common cause of acute eczema relapses. The three golden rules for reducing stress are: take regular relaxation; balance your life; and avoid bad habits.

Points to remember

1   Stick to your treatment plan for emollients and steroids, even if your skin is getting much better. Give time for hidden healing. The Combined Approach works by providing all three levels of treatment together.

2   Carry on doing Habit Reversal, concentrating especially on focus times, until you have eliminated both habit scratching and itch-response scratching.

3   Each treatment level is discontinued when the skin no longer needs it: Habit Reversal when scratching has stopped (just beyond the Look Good Point); steroid treatment when hidden healing is complete; emollients may continue to be applied at a lower frequency.

4   Catch acute eczema relapses early. Treat dryness and roughness with extra emollient applications. Treat redness and itchiness with the topical steroid twice a day for three days, then once a day for three days, then stop.

5   Stress is a common cause of acute eczema relapses. The three golden rules for reducing stress: take regular relaxation; balance your life; avoid bad habits.

chapter eight
LIVING WITHOUT ECZEMA

*I used to hate going to the beach – people always wanted you
to swim, and I had to take a big bottle of water to rinse in
and all these creams. Now I just dive into the water.*

What a novelty to start a new chapter without a homework
session! This is because you have now reached the end of the
programme, so there are no more set reviews of your progress.
However, don't let this stop you from continuing to log your
(rapidly diminishing) scratching, or from filling in the eczema and
scratching charts and body maps. You might find it useful to carry
on doing this for as long as you are moving down the healing
curve, until every bit of skin gets past the Look Good Point.
Reaching the end of the book doesn't mean stopping the
programme, it just means you have learnt all the techniques. Keep
doing the Combined Approach until you have the skin you want
– you may already be there, or you may need a little more time.

The convalescent phase
If you carry on as you have been doing, using Habit Reversal,
self-prescriptions and focus times to eliminate scratching, backed

The pattern of eczema and the healing process

Before you started the programme you had a base of chronic eczema, with acute eczema making it periodically worse. When you start the Combined Approach you use Habit Reversal to get rid of the chronic eczema, and emollient and steroid therapy to get rid of the acute eczema. As you progress down the healing curve both types of eczema clear away, first visibly clearing (obvious healing) and then going through hidden healing. During the convalescent phase your skin will still be settling down and prone to flare-ups of acute eczema, which will gradually become smaller and further apart as your skin gets stronger.

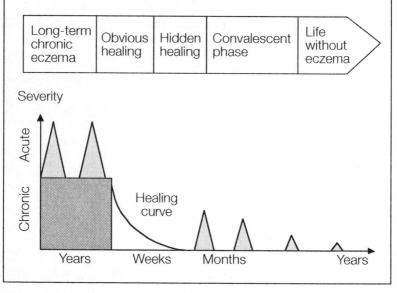

Long-term chronic eczema	Obvious healing	Hidden healing	Convalescent phase	Life without eczema

up with strict treatment plans for emollients and steroids, your chronic eczema will clear completely. Bit by bit, all the difficult areas will reach the Look Good Point and go through the two-week period of hidden healing. Now you enter the third phase of healing: the convalescent phase.

During the first three months or so after your skin has cleared, it will still be settling down. If you have suffered from severe chronic eczema for a long time your skin will be more used to being disrupted and hypersensitive than to being robust and healthy. During the convalescent phase your skin will still be quite sensitive, and it will be relatively easy to trigger a relapse. As time goes by your skin will get more resilient. It will become more and more tolerant of conditions which you would expect to provoke a flare-up, and the acute eczema blips will get smaller and further apart. As you are atopic you may always be susceptible to acute eczema flare-ups, but after the convalescent phase your skin will be much stronger. You will learn what new activities you can enjoy without problems, and which situations you still need to be careful with. For example, you may find that during the convalescent phase your skin may become strong enough not to be irritated by your favourite wool sweater, even though it still made you itch immediately after hidden healing.

Remember:

During the convalescent phase your skin is settling down, becoming less sensitive and more tolerant. Be extra-vigilant for relapses during the first three months.

Complete healing

Here's a story you might find amusing. A woman I know had dreadful eczema that made her life a misery and ruined her health for more than ten years. She swore that she would do anything, no matter how difficult or protracted, to get better.

When she started the Combined Approach her skin cleared and she thought it was a miracle. Within weeks her skin was better than it had been for a decade. From having been covered from head to toe there were just a few patches left – she was nearly at her dream of perfect skin. And then, something odd happened. She stopped trying to clear the last bit. She felt that it would be pushing her luck to aim for totally clear skin, when she was already so much better then she ever thought she could be. And after using scratching as a stress relief technique for years she found she missed it – nothing else could quite expel frustration in the same way. She thought she could be satisfied with almost clear skin, rather than completely clear skin.

What do you think? Is she silly? Deluded? A realist? It probably comes as no surprise to you that this was my story! If someone had suggested to me that I didn't want to get better I would probably have wanted to kill them. How dare they patronize me; of course I wanted to get better – how could anyone want to carry on with the pain and misery of chronic eczema if they didn't have to? But I found out that on some odd, subconscious level it was easier to get almost better than completely better. And I was not alone!

Here are some reasons for not going for complete healing:

- ❏ If it is that easy to get rid of, all my years of suffering will have been for nothing.
- ❏ I need to be able to scratch sometimes.
- ❏ It's so good already, it seems ungrateful to want more.
- ❏ I won't have an excuse for failure anymore.
- ❏ I can't concentrate on Habit Reversal forever – I want to get on with my life.

❏ I won't get any more sympathy and support from my family.

❏ I'm used to having eczema – it's part of my identity.

If your skin still has some way to go before the Look Good Point, you may be reading this with a sense of disbelief. How could anyone who knows how to get perfect skin not reach out and take it? But if your skin is almost clear you may have experienced some of these feelings. In fact, the doctors who run this programme find that it is quite common.

If you have had eczema for a very long time you may be so used to seeing yourself as someone who copes with bad eczema that it is hard to see yourself as anything else. You can't really and truly envisage yourself with clear skin. You can *dream* about it, yes, but you can't *expect* it to happen, say, in the next three weeks.

If you have struggled for years with the misery of eczema, just being able to clear it in a matter of weeks can be curiously undermining. What was the point of all those years of suffering? All those people saying how brave you were, all the money on alternative therapies that didn't work, all the experiences that were spoiled for you or that you missed altogether – they are all devalued if you can be healed so easily. The thing to remember here is that you are not being healed 'so easily'. You are adopting a whole new behaviour pattern, and having to relearn some of your most basic instincts. You have had to work really hard to get to this point.

Maybe the biggest reason for not going for complete healing is the most mundane one – a feeling that almost there is good enough. After all, the difference between totally clear skin and almost-clear-apart-from-these-bits-on-my-wrists skin is tiny, compared to the difference between either of them and all-over chronic eczema. How much difference does it really make? You're thrilled, you can wear the clothes, do the activities, and have the lifestyle you've been denied; so what about a few little patches?

Complete healing is the aim of the treatment for sound medical objectives. Here are three big reasons for going for clear skin:

1 **If you have a little bit of eczema, you will always be using steroids.**

As long as you are using steroids you are running the risk of side-effects. Using them sensibly, when your skin is inflamed, and in a way designed to minimize the amount that you have to apply, will not do you any harm. But drifting back into the old pattern of indefinite steroid applications to chronic eczema that is not being cleared is not sensible. And if you stop them while your skin is still inflamed your eczema gets worse. The only way out is complete healing.

2 **If the skin doesn't clear completely, you continue to have a significant vulnerability factor: damaged skin. This increases your chance of acute relapses.**

If you have some patches of eczema your skin stays in a sensitive, unstable state. It doesn't have the chance of an uninterrupted healing and strengthening period. Without complete healing, your skin will be much more likely to flare up.

3 **You'll never get that feel-good feeling!**

Achieving completely clear skin, and being free from eczema, maybe for the first time in years, gives you a huge boost! You really have gained complete control. You are no longer the victim but the manager. You can do anything if you can live without eczema!

Remember:

Hold out for complete healing. Allowing a few old friendly patches of eczema to remain means you'll always use steroids, always have flare-ups, and never get that feel-good factor.

Living without eczema

The aim of this whole programme, and probably your intention when you bought the book, is for you to live without eczema. Once you're through the convalescent phase, you'll be doing just that. This does not mean, however, that you should forget all about eczema. It will never be the energy-draining obsession that it once was, but you do have to make a small investment to make sure that your skin stays clear. I think you'll find it is worth it, for a life without eczema.

VIGILANCE AND THE ZAP PACK

We saw earlier that the key to preventing acute eczema relapses is to catch them right at the start. You need to be vigilant about checking for signs of a flare-up. You also need to have a fully equipped Zap Pack ready at all times. The Zap Pack is your first-aid kit – it contains the emollients and effective topical steroids that you will apply when you see the early signs of a flare-up. You will need the thickest emollient you find comfortable to use, and a stock of the topical steroids you were using for Level 2 Treatment, including all the different formulations for different areas of the body, for example, scalp, face and body steroids. It will do

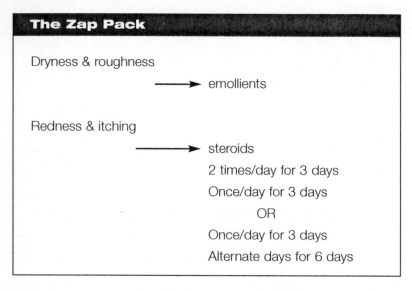

The Zap Pack

Dryness & roughness

⟶ emollients

Redness & itching

⟶ steroids
2 times/day for 3 days
Once/day for 3 days
OR
Once/day for 3 days
Alternate days for 6 days

no good to wait until your skin begins to flare up and then go to the doctor for the medicines. To stop the blip in its tracks you need to start treatment straight away, which means you always need a Zap Pack, even if your skin has been clear for months. You need to organize this with your doctor.

Remember:

Have a Zap Pack of your favourite emollients (for example, one light, one heavy duty) and topical steroids for different parts of your body ready to zap relapses before they start.

REFRESHER COURSES

If you have achieved complete healing you have successfully completed Habit Reversal, and unlearned habitual scratching behaviour. As time goes by, and all the self-prescriptions and replacement behaviours are no longer at the forefront of your mind, you may benefit from the occasional refresher course. If you have gone through a stressful time at work or some upheaval that puts strain on your skin, this is an especially good idea.

Sometimes a relapse can come at a bad time, when you are preoccupied with other things and don't feel you have enough time to give your skin the attention it needs. Under these circumstances you might even find yourself using your skin as a stress-control technique, and slipping back into habitual scratching. You really don't want this to happen.

If you find a relapse doesn't clear up with the standard approach, and is still present after a couple of weeks, then you should definitely give a refresher course a go, as a little bit of scratching may have crept back. You know the drill by now. Give yourself three days of registration (logging your scratches and noting the daily totals), and a week of Habit Reversal. This should be enough to bring everything under control again.

Remember:

From time to time you may benefit from doing a refresher course of a week's Habit Reversal.

IF THINGS GO WRONG: WHEN TO SEE YOUR DOCTOR

Of course, if ever your skin flares up abnormally badly, and does not recover with Levels 1 and 2 Treatment even though you are not scratching, go to the doctor. You may have an infection or an allergy that needs specific attention. If you get a rash that looks different from a blip of acute eczema you should also go. As your skin gets better you will be far less prone to infections, and your improving general health will make you less sensitive to allergens, but you should still be careful with your skin.

QUALITY OF LIFE

Think of all the things that having chronic eczema used to spoil. Long list, isn't it? These are all the things that are better when you can live without eczema. Just about every area of your world improves. Your quality of life skyrockets when you live without eczema. This has probably been your motivator all the way through the programme – it certainly was mine.

The first things to improve tend to be your moods, your sleep patterns, and your self-confidence. You start to have a feeling of general well-being. You can wear a wider range of clothes, do more sports and activities, and you feel all sorts of social restraints being lifted. Relationships tend to become much easier, with friends and with partners. Close friends and family who have cared for you while your eczema was bad feel relieved and relaxed about your skin as they shed their perceived responsibility. At work, school, college or running the home, you have more energy, can accept more responsibility, and concentrate better. All this is over and above the bliss of being free from the pain, the inconvenience, and the exhaustion of living with chronic eczema.

Living without eczema is wonderful – and now you can do it. Good luck!

Points to remember

1 During the convalescent phase your skin is settling down, becoming less sensitive and more tolerant. Be extra-vigilant for relapses during the first three months.

2 Hold out for complete healing. Allowing a few old friendly patches of eczema to remain means you'll always use steroids, always have flare-ups, and never get that feel-good factor.

3 Have a Zap Pack of your favourite emollients and topical steroids for different parts of your body ready to zap relapses before they start.

Helen is a residential negotiator, and has had atopic eczema since infancy. Now 37, she completed the programme two years ago. Thinking back to living with eczema, she says the worst thing was feeling embarrassed about how she looked. Her job involves dealing with the public all the time, and having eczema on her face and hands made her feel awkward at work and socially. 'People used to ask me if I had a black eye', she remembers. But since mastering Habit Reversal, her skin has cleared completely. 'I get patches appearing between my fingers if I get stressed, but the Zap Pack (see page 86) soon gets rid of them.' The best thing about being clear, she says, is feeling comfortable about meeting people, and not rubbing her eyes all the time anymore.

chapter nine
FREQUENTLY ASKED QUESTIONS

You almost enjoy scratching, and think 'Hah, take that!' as you're doing it – it's as if you're taking revenge on your skin. You're not attractive anyway so it doesn't matter.

WHAT IS ECZEMA?

Eczema is a group of skin conditions, sometimes also called dermatitis. It is characterized by dry, itchy skin, which can become raw and bleeding when it is severe. The name 'eczema' comes from the Greek word *ekzein*, which means 'to boil over', probably because of the hot, angry surface of eczematous skin.

WHAT ARE THE DIFFERENT TYPES OF ECZEMA?

There are several different types of eczema. Although they can look similar, they may have different causes and treatments, and it is important to be sure which one you have. If in any doubt, go to your doctor for a diagnosis.

Atopic eczema: This is the commonest type of eczema, and the subject of this book. It is characterized by a dry, itchy skin condition, often starting before the age of two years, and usually in the form of a visible rash. In infants, the rash often appears on the cheeks, in children and adults it usually starts in skin folds (inside elbows, backs of knees, under the neck, fronts of ankles). It tends to become chronic on exposed areas, like the hands and face. The skin is often red and hot, and the itching can be very intense. The skin is frequently dry, even when it is not inflamed. The condition tends to run in families, and people with atopic eczema often also suffer from hay fever, asthma or both. The rash may flare up and calm down at different times.

Contact dermatitis. This occurs when the skin comes into contact with something which triggers a reaction. This type of eczema can be divided into **irritant contact dermatitis**, where frequent contact with something irritates the skin (for example detergents or chemicals) and **allergic contact dermatitis**, where the skin reacts to something to which you are allergic (for example, nickel or rubber). In both cases, the reaction may happen after being repeatedly exposed to the irritant or allergen, and the best course of action is to protect your skin by avoiding the substance in future.

Seborrhoeic eczema: In babies, this appears as the well-known cradle cap or starts in the nappy area. It is quite common, and the exact cause is not understood. It usually clears up after a few months, and does not appear to cause the baby any discomfort (although it might upset the proud parents). In adults, seborrhoeic eczema is associated with natural oily secretions from the skin. It usually occurs as dry, flaky skin (dandruff) on the scalp, and can spread to the face and chest. It is sometimes treated with an anti-fungal cream.

Varicose (or gravitational) eczema: This is associated with poor circulation, and usually occurs on the lower legs of older people.

The skin breaks out in an itchy, inflamed rash, and can develop a speckled appearance. If it is not treated (usually with emollients and sometimes steroids), it can worsen into an ulcer.

Discoid eczema: This appears as round patches of reddened skin (hence the name), which can get itchy and weepy. The patches are mostly distributed on the trunk and legs, and the condition is treated with emollients and sometimes steroids.

WHAT IS ATOPY?

Atopy literally means 'strange disease', and it is a description for a variable group of symptoms, rather than one defined set. People with atopy have excessive immune reactions to factors which affect others much less, making them prone to eczema, asthma and hay fever. Atopy is thought to be hereditary. About 25–30 per cent of the population is atopic.

HOW MANY PEOPLE HAVE ATOPIC ECZEMA?

Since the condition varies from mild to severe and not everybody with eczema is under the care of a doctor, it is hard to say exactly how many people have it. But around 5–15 per cent of school children have eczema, and 2–10 per cent of adults.

ARE MORE PEOPLE GETTING ECZEMA, ASTHMA AND HAY FEVER?

It's hard to tell, but it seems likely. Studies are showing that more people are showing signs of atopy, with associated conditions of eczema, asthma and hay fever. Possible explanations for this include a higher level of exposure to allergens such as house dust mite droppings, associated with centrally-heated and carpeted houses, or slower immune system development in children who are not exposed to dirt as much as previous generations. However, there is no proven cause.

WHAT CAUSES ATOPIC ECZEMA?

There is no single cause for eczema. Atopic people are more likely to be sensitive to environmental factors than other people, triggering extreme immune system reactions which affect their skin. The skin reacts by becoming inflamed, itchy and dry. This starts the itch-scratch-itch cycle, where skin is continually being damaged by scratching, prolonging and worsening the inflammation, and eventually leading to chronic eczema.

WHAT'S THE DIFFERENCE BETWEEN CHRONIC AND ACUTE ATOPIC ECZEMA?

Acute eczema is eczema that flares up in response to a trigger. The skin becomes inflamed, red and dry. It can be treated effectively with emollients and steroids, and will die down within a few days.

Chronic eczema is eczema that remains the same week on week, and doesn't clear. It is caused by constantly damaging the skin with acute eczema by scratching it, so that the skin never gets a chance to heal. Chronic eczema needs to be treated by changing the behaviour, removing the scratching so that the steroids and emollients have a chance to work.

IS THERE A CURE FOR ATOPIC ECZEMA?

There is a cure for chronic atopic eczema. The cure involves changing your behaviour, stopping your habitual scratching and allowing the other conventional treatments (steroids and emollients) a chance to work. Remember, though, that there is no cure for atopy, which is a condition that you will always have. This means that you will always be prone to new flare-ups of eczema in response to a trigger, but these can be controlled quickly and easily.

IS ECZEMA CONTAGIOUS?

No. You can't catch eczema from someone, or give eczema to another person. The condition is caused by your own skin's reactions, and not by infection from someone else. But eczema can become infected by other contagious conditions (see below).

WHAT HAPPENS IF MY ECZEMA IS INFECTED?

Skin with eczema can be prone to infections, because the damaged skin surface is less able to defend against them. Various bacteria, viruses and fungi can infect skin. If eczematous skin gets infected, it may crack and weep, becoming wet all the time. It may also get redder and more painful, and may develop sores or spots. If you think your eczema may be infected, see your doctor immediately.

DO CHILDREN GROW OUT OF ECZEMA?

Most children do grow out of eczema, with between two thirds and three quarters becoming free of it by their mid-teens.

WILL MY CHILD GET ECZEMA IF I HAVE IT?

Not necessarily. A combination of genetic and environmental factors are thought to influence which people get eczema, and parents do not always pass the condition on to their children.

WHAT ARE THE MAIN TREATMENTS FOR ECZEMA?
The main conventional treatments for eczema are emollients and steroids.

Emollients, or moisturizers, help to treat the dryness that characterizes skin with eczema. They don't add moisture directly to the skin. Rather, they act as a barrier over the skin's surface, preventing moisture from evaporating. This is necessary because eczema disrupts the skin's surface and damages its natural waterproofing abilities, letting it dry out too quickly.

Steroids are drugs which reduce the inflammation of eczematous skin. They are usually prescribed as topical steroids, which means they are applied straight onto the skin in a cream or ointment. Topical steroids come in four different strengths: mild, moderate, potent and very potent, which are prescribed according to the area of the body which needs to be treated and the severity of the eczema. In very severe cases, steroids can be given in pills or injections.

The new treatment for eczema, described in this book, treats the third aspect of eczema – *scratching*. For successful treatment, the scratching, the inflammation and the dryness all need to be addressed together.

WHAT ABOUT COMPLEMENTARY THERAPIES?
Complementary therapies cover a huge range of different treatments, many of which claim to offer a holistic treatment for the whole person, rather than just the skin. There has been very little research into the effectiveness of different approaches, although there is anecdotal evidence that people find them helpful. Many complementary therapies can be used alongside conventional treatments. The safest approach is to discuss them with your

doctor, make sure any complementary practitioners are suitably qualified, and avoid abandoning your conventional treatments suddenly in favour of a new idea.

IS STRESS CAUSING MY ECZEMA?

Stress is a common trigger for acute eczema flare-ups. But it isn't causing your chronic eczema – or at least not directly. Chronic eczema is caused by habitual scratching, which may itself be made worse by stress. If you think stress is a big factor in your eczema… you are probably right.

WHAT CAN I DO TO STOP MY SKIN FROM ITCHING?

The itchiness of eczema is one of its most distressing symptoms. You can help reduce it by never letting your skin get dry – always apply emollients before it feels like you need to. Keep your skin cool and allow it to breath by using cotton sheets and clothing – wool and synthetic fabrics can irritate and overheat it.

appendix one
TOPICAL CORTICOSTEROIDS IN COMMON USE*

GRADE IV: MILD
Hydrocortisone 0.5% cream/ointment
Hydrocortisone 1% cream/ointment
Hydrocortisone 2.5% cream/ointment

GRADE III: MODERATE
Eumovate cream/ointment (clobetastone butyrate 0.05%)
Alphaderm cream (Hydrocortisone 1%, urea 10%)

GRADE II: POTENT
Betnovate cream/ointment/scalp application
   (betamethasone [as valerate] 0.1%)
Cutivate cream (flutisone propionate 0.05%)
Cutivate ointment (flutisone propionate 0.005%)
Diprosone cream/ointment (betamethasone 0.05%
   [as dipropionate])

---

* List of steroids from Bridgett C, Noren P & Staughton R. (1996) *Atopic Skin Disease: A manual for practitioners*. Wrightson Biomedical Publishing.

Elocon cream/ointment (mometasone furoate 0.1%)

Locoid cream (hydrocortisone butyrate 0.1%)

Metosyn cream/ointment/scalp lotion (fluocinonide 0.05%)

Nerisone oily cream (diflucortolone valerate 0.1%)

Propaderm cream/ointment (beclomethasone dipropionate 0.025%)

Synalar cream/ointment/scalp gel (fluocinolone acetonide 0.015%)

GRADE I: VERY POTENT

Dermovate cream/ointment/scalp application (clobetasol propionate 0.05%)

Nerisone forte oily cream (diflucortolone valerate 0.3%)

appendix two
WORKBOOK

CHART I: REGISTRATION

Record the number of times you scratch using your hand logger, every day for seven days. Remember: Do not try to avoid scratching. Allow registration to make you more aware of when it happens. Scratching = rubbing = picking = touching.

Date							
Total scratches							
Times when I scratched most today							
1							
2							
3							
4							
5							
Percentage of scratching coming from itch							
%							

CHART 2: HISTORY OF ECZEMA

Question	Ring or fill in your answer
At what age did you first develop eczema?	< 6 months; < 1 year; < 3 years; 3-5 years; 6-11 years; 12-18 years; >18 years
How bad was your eczema as a child?	Mild; moderate; severe
Were you hospitalized for your eczema?	Once; 2-5 times; over 5 times
What was the impact of your eczema on your family, as a child?	Mild; moderate; severe
What parts of your body were mainly affected in childhood?	
What happened to your eczema in childhood?	Cleared and came back Always there
Did you have problems at school because of eczema?	

Did you have time off school because of your eczema?	None; a little; a lot
Did you ever attend eczema summer camps or holidays?	
Did your eczema change during adolescence?	Different rash Different distribution Different symptoms
Did your eczema go away in adolescence?	
Now, are you ever completely free of eczema?	
If not, when were you last completely free?	
If so, how long are you free from eczema?	Months; weeks; days at a time
Is your eczema making your life a misery?	If so, for months; weeks; days at a time
Where are you relative to your eczema?	Victim/ Out of control Managing/ In control ← ——————————→

What parts of your body are mainly affected?	Scalp; face; neck; arms; hands; chest; back; abdomen; legs; feet
When your eczema is bad, how long is it bad for?	Days; weeks; months
When your eczema is better, how long is it better for?	Days; weeks; months
About how often do bad/new episodes occur?	____ times per month ____ times per year
Do you think you are allergic:	To foods; animals; house dust mite; other_____
Does anything make your eczema better?	Holidays; relaxation; weather; season; other_____
Does anything make your eczema worse?	Stress; emotion; weather; season; alcohol; menstrual cycle; central heating; air conditioning; exercise; water hardness; other_____
Do you have/have you had: asthma?	None; mild; moderate; severe
Do you have/have you had: hay fever?	None; mild; moderate; severe

CHART 3: ECZEMA REVIEW

Estimate scores in each category for the past few days

	Week 1	Week 3	Week 5	Week 7	Week 9
Date					
1 How bad is your eczema overall on a scale of 0-10: 10 = worst ever; 0 = perfect skin					
2 What percentage of your eczema is old, as opposed to new? New = appeared in past 10 days					
3 Where is the worst eczema? Where is the rest?					
4 What percentage of your scratching is coming from itch?					

CHART 4: BODY MAP

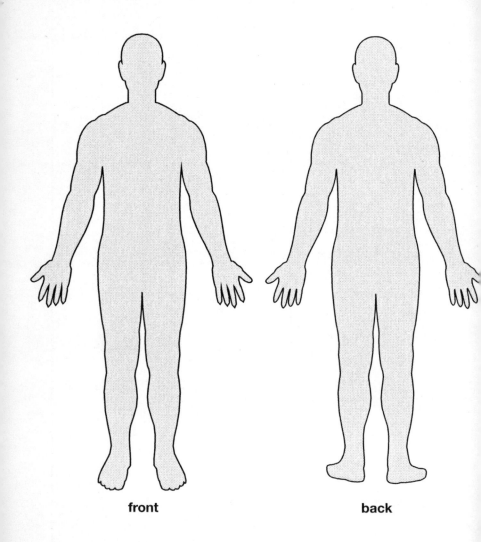

front   back

CHART 5: LEVELS 1 & 2 TREATMENT PLAN

Level 1: Dry skin.

Treatment: emollients   Date:

Emollients	Apply where	Apply when
1.		
2.		
3.		

BE CONSISTENT!

Level 2: Eczema and itch

Treatment: steroids

<u>Steroid 1</u>

Name:

To be applied where:

Date							
a.m.							
p.m.							

Date							
a.m.							
p.m.							

<u>Steroid 2</u>

Name:

To be applied where:

Date							
a.m.							
p.m.							

Date							
a.m.							
p.m.							

DON'T STOP TOO SOON!

CHART 6: HABIT REVERSAL

CLENCH... COUNT... SOMETHING NICE... PRESS

Continue registration to measure your progress:

Date								% from itch
No. scratches								

Date								% from itch
No. scratches								

Date								% from itch
No. scratches								

Date								% from itch
No. scratches								

Date								% from itch
No. scratches								

Date								% from itch
No. scratches								

PREPARE YOURSELF
DO IT QUICKLY
KEEP HANDS BUSY

Difficult situations

Dispense with:	Otherwise – Self-prescription:
1.	1.
2.	2.
3.	3.
4.	4.
5.	5.
6.	6.
7.	7.
8.	8.
9.	9.
10.	10.

CHART 6: HABIT REVERSAL - CONTINED

Date								% from itch
No. scratches								

Date								% from itch
No. scratches								

Date								% from itch
No. scratches								

Date								% from itch
No. scratches								

Date								% from itch
No. scratches								

Date								% from itch
No. scratches								

Date								% from itch
No. scratches								

CHART 7: FOCUS TIMES FOR
ANTI-SCRATCHING BEHAVIOUR

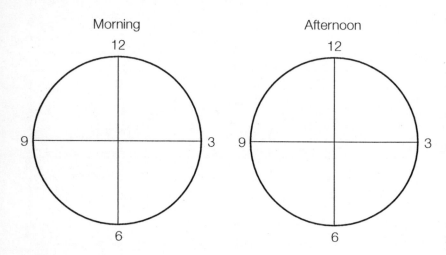

Focus times

Times	Circumstances	Self-prescription
1		
2		
3		
4		

Dear Doctor,

HABIT REVERSAL PROGRAMME FOR CHRONIC ATOPIC ECZEMA

Your patient, ..., is starting a self-help programme designed to treat chronic atopic eczema. This approach is a version of the Habit Reversal programme developed by Drs Bridgett and Staughton at the Dermatology Department at Chelsea and Westminster Hospital in London. The self-help programme is set out in *The Eczema Solution*, published by Vermilion.

Your patient will follow a course of exercises, which aim to identify and reduce the scratching behaviour that always plays a significant role in chronic atopic eczema. These exercises are not designed to replace conventional treatments. Your patient will benefit from regular reviews of their steroid, emollient and other treatments as they go through the programme.

Your patient has made an appointment on .... (date) to discuss their current and future treatment needs with you. They will have read about the importance of preventing skin from drying with emollients (rather than allowing skin to become dry and then applying emollients). They will have read about treating eczematous skin with topical steroids, about the necessity to use a drug which is potent enough to be effective in treating their eczema, and about the importance of continuing to apply the steroid until healing is complete. Experience with patients going through the programme under the supervision of Chelsea and Westminster Dermatology Department showed that at the start, relatively severe eczema benefited from treatment with a higher potency steroid, which could then be discontinued as the eczema improved. This may result in a lower overall steroid application than using a less potent steroid for an indefinite period, thus helping to allay some patients' concerns about using strong treatments.

Your patient has also been encouraged to discuss their mental state with you, including any problems with anxiety or stress. These may be linked to eczema and could affect their ability to complete the programme.

As your patient proceeds through the programme, they will learn when and why they scratch, and techniques to reduce and then change their scratching behaviour. This aims to remove the constant damaging behaviour which leads to chronic eczema. However, it does not represent a 'cure' for atopy, and your patient will need to remain vigilant for flare-ups of acute eczema, and be prepared to treat them immediately with emollients and steroids.

This information sheet is intended to provide you with a brief explanation of the programme, so that you and your patient will be able to work together to tackle chronic eczema. For more information, please see the information sources below.

Yours sincerely,
Sue Armstrong-Brown

Armstrong Brown, S. (2002) *The Eczema Solution*. Vermilion.
Bridgett C, Noren P & Staughton R. (1996) *Atopic Skin Disease: A manual for practitioners*. Wrightson Biomedical Publishing.

index

acute eczema, 12, 28, 67, 93
see also relapses
alcohol, 42, 77
allergens, atopy, 10–11, 92–3
allergic contact dermatitis, 91
Alphaderm cream, 97
alternative therapies, 5–16, 95–6
anxiety, 42
asthma, 4, 10–11, 92
atopic eczema, 11, 90–1
see also eczema
atopy, 10–11, 92
attitudes to eczema, 40–3, 81–5

babies
atopic eczema, 90–1
seborrhoeic eczema, 91
balanced life, 76–7
bath additives, 35
beclomethasone dipropionate, 98
behaviour
distribution of scratching, 61–4, 110
frequency of scratching, 59, 69
Habit Reversal, 46–55, 59–61, 107–9
Besnier's prurigo, 2
betamethasone, 97
Betnovate cream, 97
blood vessels
eczematous skin, 13
varicose eczema, 91–2
body map, 29, 57, 104
Bridgett, Chris, 2

caffeine, 77
cells, eczematous skin, 13–14
Chelsea and Westminster Hospital, London, 2, 9

children
atopic eczema, 90–1
growing out of eczema, 94
inheritance of eczema, 94
seborrhoeic eczema, 91
Chinese herbs, 5–6
chronic eczema, 12–16, 28, 67, 93
circulation problems, varicose eczema, 3, 91–2
clobetasol propionate, 98
clobetastone butyrate, 97
coffee, 77
cold sore virus, 4–5
Combined Approach, 17
complete healing, 81–5
complimentary therapies, 5–6, 95–6
contact dermatitis, 91
convalescent phase, 79–81
corticosteroids *see* steroids
counters, logging scratching, 20–4
cradle cap, 91
creams, 35–6
Cutivate, 97

dandruff, 91
danger times, scratching, 51–3
depression, 42
dermatitis *see* eczema
dermatologists, 32
dermis, healing, 39–40
Dermovate, 98
diagnosis, 11
diet, 77
diflucortolone valerate, 98
Diprosone, 97
discoid eczema, 3, 92
distribution of eczema, 29, 57, 67
doctors, 32–3, 43, 111–12
doodling, 52
drugs *see* steroids
dry skin, 13

emollients, 16, 33–7, 58, 68

eczema
acute eczema, 12, 28, 67, 93
causes, 93
chronic eczema, 12–16, 28, 67, 93
complete healing, 81–5
convalescent phase, 79–81
diagnosis, 11
distribution, 29, 57, 67
incidence of, 10, 92
living without, 85–8
relapses, 72–8
severity scale, 28, 57, 67, 103
types of, 3, 90–2
eczema herpeticum, 4–5
eczematous skin, 13–15
Elocon cream, 98
emollients, 16, 32–7, 58, 68, 95
applying, 34–5, 58
relapses, 74
stopping, 72
types of, 35–6
Zap Pack, 85–6
epidermis, healing, 39–40
Eumovate cream, 97
exercise, 76

flare-ups *see* relapses
fluocinolone acetonide, 98
fluocinonide, 98
focus times, scratching, 61–4, 110
food, 77
Francis of Assisi, St, 77

genetics, 94
GPs, 32–3, 43, 111–12
gravitational eczema, 3, 91–2

Habit Reversal, 17, 46–55, 59–61, 107

refresher courses, 86–7
stopping, 70–1
habitual scratching, 15–16,
17
hand tally counters, 20–4
hands, Habit Reversal,
52–3
hay fever, 4, 11, 92
healing
complete healing, 81-5
healing curve, 70–2
hidden healing, 39–40, 58
itching and, 69
Look Good Point, 39–40,
58, 74
Helen, 65
history of eczema, 27,
100–2
homeopathy, 5–6
hydrocortisone, 97, 98

immune system, atopy,
92–3
infections, 4–5, 87, 94
insomnia, 42
intra-muscular steroids, 37
irritant contact dermatitis,
91
itching, 14, 96
and healing, 69
percentage of scratching
coming from, 29–30,
59–60

Laura, 45
lichenified skin, 14–15
Locoid cream, 98
logging scratching, 20–4,
99
Look Good Point, healing,
39–40, 58, 74
mental state, 40–3
complete healing, 81–5
Metosyn cream, 98
moisture loss, emollients,
33–4
moisturizers see emollients
mometasone furoate, 98

National Eczema Society, 4
Nerisone forte oily cream,
98

Nerisone oily cream, 98
new eczema, 28–9, 57
Noren, Dr Peter, 2

occupational eczema, 3
ointments, 35–6
old eczema, 28–9, 57, 67
older people, varicose
eczema, 3, 91–2
oral steroids, 37

personal history, 27, 100–2
phobias, 42
Propaderm, 98

quality of life, 88

recording scratching, 24–6,
99
reflexology, 6
refresher courses, relapses,
86–7
Reggie, 19
relapses, 72–8
refresher courses, 86–7
stress and, 75–8
Zap Pack, 85–6
relationships, 88
relaxation, 76

scalp oil, 35
scratching
ABC of, 47
danger times, 51–3
focus times, 61–4, 110
frequency, 59, 69
Habit Reversal, 46–55,
59–61, 107–9
habitual scratching,
15–16, 17
lichenification of skin,
14–15
logging, 20–4, 99
losing habit, 70–1
percentage coming from
itch, 29–30, 59–60
recording, 24–6, 99
relapses, 73, 86–7
stopping, 16–17
techniques of, 15, 59
troubleshooting, 60–1
seborrheic eczema, 3, 91

self-monitoring, 27
self-prescription, Habit
Reversal, 53–4
serenity prayer, 77
side-effects, steroids, 37–8
skin
convalescent phase, 79–81
distribution of eczema,
29, 57, 67
dryness, 13
eczematous skin, 13–14
emollients, 33–7, 58, 68,
95
healing, 39–40, 58, 69
infections, 4–5, 87, 94
itching, 96
lichenification, 14–15
stopping emollients, 72
washing, 36
sleep, 42, 77
sleeping pills, 77
smoking, 77
soap substitutes, 35, 36
Staughton, Dr Richard, 2
steroids, 32–3, 37–40, 58,
69, 95
applying, 38
long-term effects, 5, 37–8
recording use, 43–4
and relapses, 73, 74
stopping, 71–2
stopping too soon,
38–40, 58
types of, 97–8
Zap Pack, 85–6
stress, 75–8, 96
Su-Lin, 9
symptoms, 11
Synalar, 98

tea, 77
telephone calls, Habit
Reversal, 52
topical steroids, 37–40, 95
tranquillizers, 77

varicose eczema, 3, 91–2
vesicles, eczematous skin,
13

washing skin, 36
Zap Pack, 85–6